STRETCHING

for

50+

STRETCHING
for
50+

**A Customized Program
for Increasing Flexibility,
Avoiding Injury and
Enjoying an Active Lifestyle**

DR. KARL KNOPF

photography by Robert Holmes

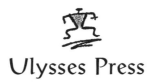

Ulysses Press

Published in the United States by
Ulysses Press
P.O. Box 3440
Berkeley, CA 94703
www.ulyssespress.com

ISBN10: 1-56975-445-4
ISBN13: 978-1-56975-445-0
Library of Congress Control Number 2004108862

Printed in Canada by Webcom

10 9 8 7 6

Editorial/Production	Ashley Chase, Lily Chou, Claire Chun, Steven Zah Schwartz
Indexer	Sayre Van Young
Design	Sarah Levin
Photography	Robert Holmes
Front cover image	© Royalty-free/Corbis
Models	Vivian Gunderson, Phyllis Ritchie, Michael O'Meara

Distributed by Publishers Group West

Please Note
This book has been written and published strictly for informational purposes, and in no way
should be used as a substitute for consultation with health care professionals. You should not
consider educational material herein to be the practice of medicine or to replace consultation
with a physician or other medical practitioner. The author and publisher are providing you
with information in this work so that you can have the knowledge and can choose, at your
own risk, to act on that knowledge. The author and publisher also urge all readers to be
aware of their health status and to consult health care professionals before beginning any
health program.

contents

part one:

getting
started

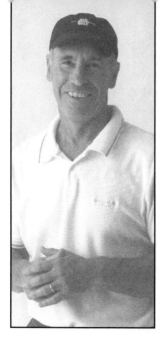

introduction

This book is designed for people who know that health and wellness are not achieved by luck but by staying active and doing as many good things for themselves (such as eating well and engaging in regular physical activity) as they can to live well for as long as possible. The decisions we make daily are the foundation of successful living.

Most of us 50-plus folks were taught by a number of outdated rules that could cause us more harm than good, including the old paradigm of more is better, which leads many of us to overdoing it. The intent of this book is to assist you to train smart, not hard.

In the '70s, fitness was all about aerobics; in the '90s, many of us started lifting weights. All this time, unfortunately, we neglected an important aspect of fitness—flexibility. Even now, we often fail to see how important flexibility is until we get hurt overdoing something, or our chiropractor or therapist tells us we have muscle imbalances (from poor posture, for example) that are manifesting themselves in chronic neck and low back pain.

I often see students who fail to see the light until it is too late. They find themselves with hunched-over posture and a head that juts forward, which makes them feel and look older than their years. I find it interesting that folks will opt for plastic surgery, yet have poor posture that makes them look like Grandma Moses. Most poor postures can be improved with regular and sensible exercise if done early on. I like the saying that most of the things that get worse with age can be positively influenced with proper exercise.

This book does not have hard and fast rules. The only rule in this book is to learn to listen to your body and heed what it says. A wise person once told me that if we watched animals, we would be less likely to get hurt when exercising, and I think he was right. Think a moment about a cat or a dog; before they get up and run, they take a moment to reach and stretch. Not because someone told them to but because it feels right. If a dog gets tired, it stops and maybe gets a drink—it listens to its body. I want us to turn inward and feel what is best for us. No one knows your body better than you! You are the captain of your ship. Everyone else is a member of your fitness crew.

Please keep these concepts in mind as you navigate the waters of the ages:

- Stretch what is tight and strengthen what is lax.
- Do unto the front as you do unto your back.
- Do unto the left as you do to the right.

I sincerely think the secret to successful aging is to stay flexible in both your mind and body.

Three things that contribute to a successful life are strength, suppleness and a sense of humor.
—Anonymous

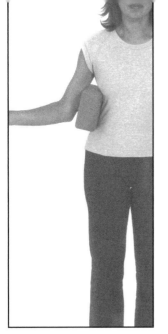

flexibility and aging

Have you ever woken up stiff and sore, or found that your shoelaces are a little farther away than they used to be, or you need help getting your dress zipper pulled up? These are the little signs that your flexibility is decreasing.

Grab the skin on the back of your hand and hold it for a moment. Does it spring right back? As we age, we lose elasticity in our skin and connective tissue. The effects of adaptive shortening of our muscles (when a muscle gets overly tight from too much work), poor body mechanics, and the misuse, disuse and abuse of our muscles and joints contribute to making us look and feel older than our years.

What Is Flexibility?

Flexibility is the range of motion (ROM) around a joint and is specific to each joint. Being able to touch your toes, for instance, doesn't mean your shoulder joint is flexible. Flexibility is influenced by many factors, two of which we have little control over: gender (women are generally more flexible than men) and the anatomical shape of our

bones and how they form to make a joint. However, we can significantly improve our flexibility by stretching regularly, which this book will help you to do.

Flexibility appears to peak, in most joints, for males around age 24 and females somewhere between the ages of 25 and 30. After that, flexibility starts to decline. While flexibility and the ability to stay flexible generally declines with age, studies have found that individuals who follow a progressive and regular stretching program are able to delay and even reverse this degeneration. I really believe that our actual age has less to do with aging than how we live and treat our bodies.

The type of physical activity that we participate in can make our muscles tight. Basically, the more muscular a person is, the more inflexible they are. When

the same muscles are used over and over again, they become stiffer. Many times we overuse, misuse and/or abuse our bodies in work or even play, which can lead to soft tissue injuries or even osteoarthritis. Joseph Pilates, the creator of Pilates, said, "The stronger the strong muscles get, the weaker the weak muscles become." This imbalance sets us up for injury, which is why stretching is so important. Overworking muscles can make us inflexible if we don't stretch, but being too sedentary may contribute to making us inflexible as well.

Importance of Flexibility

Flexibility is considered an important aspect of a total body fitness program. Unfortunately, we often neglect this part of our workout in favor of aerobics and strength training; most of us who want to look and be fit often overlook stretching in lieu of a few more minutes on the exercise cycle or a few more repetitions with the weights. If we do stretch, it is just a quick series of bouncing toe touches or a few windmills. Very often, improper stretching causes more harm than good.

As we age, our ability to maintain independence through functional mobility is of utmost importance. Flexibility of our muscles and joints dictates our ability to perform our daily activities and avoid injury. Proper flexibility plays a significant part in how we stand, how we walk and even our ability to maintain balance. Balance, in its various guises, is one key to successful aging. This includes keeping your mind balanced with mental stimulation, keeping your center of gravity balanced so you don't fall, and keeping your body balanced by strengthening weak muscles and stretching tight muscles.

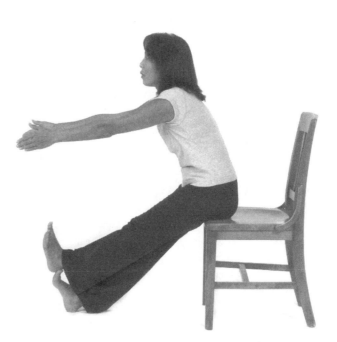

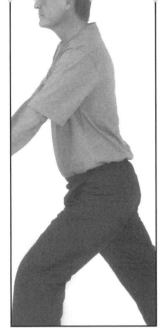

benefits of stretching

Many of us over 50 years of age often complain of stiffness. A comprehensive stretching program will help us release muscle tension and soreness, as well as reduce the risk of injury. Just spending a few minutes a day to stretch will assist in preventing soft tissue trauma such as muscle strains and ligament injuries.

Enhanced flexibility also fosters greater body awareness, which leads to an improved connection between the mind and the body. A good relationship between the mind and our muscles allows us a better ability to move our joints within their natural ranges of motion. Keep in mind that the more efficient your movements are, the more easily daily tasks can be performed. Overly tight muscles can restrict full motion in and around a joint. This tightness can limit everything from your tennis serve to walking.

Generally, poor flexibility and decreased joint range can be restored more easily if addressed early on, before it becomes a chronic problem. The longer the inflexibility exists, the more difficult it is to restore and the

more likely it will become permanent. When muscles are flexible, joints can align themselves in the biomechanical manner in which they were designed. This results in improvement in everything from our ability to move, our posture and just being able to breathe more completely.

It is easy to understand why flexibility training is short-changed. Unlike cardiovascular training that improves our heart function and assists in weight control, or strength training that improves our appearance, fosters bone density and may even improve functional fitness, stretching just seems to be a perfunctory duty. While stretching may not reduce long-term health risks, it does improve posture and our quality of life.

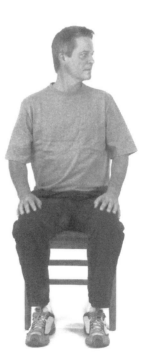

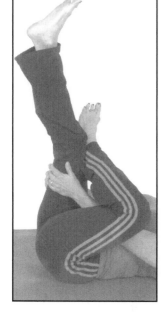

tune in to your body

As we get older, our body recovers more slowly from various physical activities. It's like a well-maintained vintage car can often run just as well as a newer sports car, but needs more TLC. The vintage car takes a little longer to warm up and needs to be tuned up more frequently, and so it is with our 50-plus bodies.

When you stretch, keep the movements controlled and maintain good posture, and also really listen to your body—especially your neck, back, shoulders and knees. When you are warming up, use this time to take inventory of your body. Heed what it says; if you feel crunches in your joints, please don't ignore them. Listen for snaps, crackles and pops—if they get louder or cause pain, see a doctor before they turn into real problems. Prevention is always cheaper than treatment, and keep in mind our vintage car analogy: it is always wiser and cheaper to do preventative maintenance than it is to do major repair work, thus physical therapy is cheaper than surgery. Remember also the two-hour rule: two hours post-exercise, you should

not feel worse than you did before you exercised. If you do, re-evaluate what you are doing.

Don't stretch:

- If you have had a recent fracture.
- If you have had a recent sprain/strain or suspect you have one.
- If you suspect that you have osteoporosis or osteopenia. Speak with your doctor about what is best for you.
- If you have pain or discomfort in a joint and around a muscle.
- If you have an infected or inflamed joint.

When in doubt, speak to your health professional.

Proper Posture

Proper posture is essential in preventing injury and muscle

imbalances. Basically, stand with your weight over the balls of your feet and heels, tuck your tailbone between your legs (imagine that you are resting on the edge of a bar stool), make the distance from your belly button and your chest as far apart as possible, and pull your belly button in and then place a imaginary apple under your chin. From a side view, your ears, shoulders and hips should be aligned (see the image on page 13). A mental picture that works for my students is to think of your body as a tube of toothpaste, with all the forces squeezing you in and upright.

When sitting, keep your ears aligned over your shoulders and your shoulders aligned over your hips; the knees are aligned over the ankles.

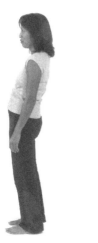
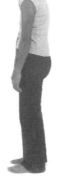
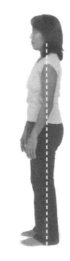

Hyperextension of back   Slouching   Proper posture!

Neck

The old expression "Don't stick your neck out" is excellent fitness advice. The neck is very fragile! Doing anything too fast or too hard can cause serious problems. Never "warm up" your neck by rolling your head around in fast circles—in fact, all quick neck movements are a bad idea. Avoid full neck circles

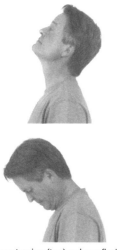

Hyperextension (top) or hyperflexion (bottom) puts undue pressure on the neck arteries.

because they strain supporting ligaments and can lead to pinched nerves. Other things to avoid include hyperflexion, when you force your chin to your chest, and hyperextension, when you arch your neck too far back. Neck extensions can also put pressure on the arteries of the neck, which can cause high blood pressure and compromise blood flow to the brain. Some women have had strokes while leaning back to get their hair washed at a salon, hence the term "beauty parlor" syndrome. The exercises in this book will show you safe and sane ways to increase the flexibility of your neck.

Low Back

Most of us will experience back pain at some time in our lives. It is critical to protect your back when you stretch. Keep your low back stable at all times. All back exercises should be done in a slow and controlled manner, and

if they increase in discomfort— STOP. Never do stretches in which you bend forward and rotate at the same time: for example, windmill toe touches are a very bad idea. Also avoid bending backward at the waist, such as in yoga stretches that call for you to raise both hands over your head and look up. Quick, uncontrolled trunk twists are not a good idea, either, because torque generated by the twisting action strains the low back. Be careful when doing fast or forced side bends, too. When sitting on the floor with your legs extended in front of you, be

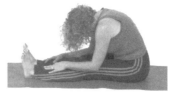

Bad: back is too rounded

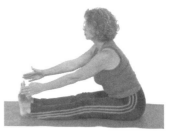

Better: back is flat but arms should be parallel to the ground

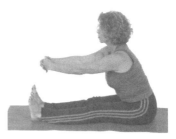

Best: proper form for reaching

sure to keep your back flat when reaching forward.

Shoulders

Shoulder problems are an increasing concern for the over-50 fitness person. Be careful when you bring your arms above your head, and always control any movement that causes you to raise your arms above shoulder height. Relax your shoulders and don't shrug when you're doing arm exercises. Try your best to keep your shoulder blades pulled together when doing arm moves as well. If your shoulders are tight, don't arch your back to make up for your inflexibility.

Knees

The knees are designed to straighten and bend; any other movement is putting them at some level of risk. The knees

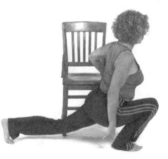

Incorrect: thigh is not parallel to floor and knee is extending beyond the toes

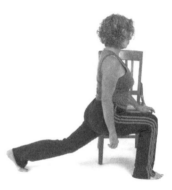

Correct: thigh is parallel to floor and knee is aligned with the ankle

and toes should always point in the same direction. Avoid any movements that make your knees rotate or twist, and never twist your body while your feet are planted on the floor. Never straighten your knee so far that it hyperextends, or overly straightens the leg. Also avoid thigh stretches like the "hurdler's stretch," which cause your knees to bend too much. Forcing your knee to bend too far over-

stretches the ligaments of the knee and can make the knee joint unstable. Avoid deep knee bends, and make sure you don't squat any lower than the point at which your thighs are parallel to the floor. Always remember: Keep your knees "soft" (that is, slightly bent) when stretching. Lastly, don't allow the knee to extend past the toes.

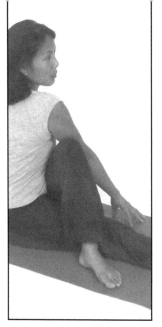

how to stretch

When stretching, always progress slowly and gently. You are unique so don't compete with anyone else or even yourself. Some days you will be pliable and some days you will be as stiff as a board—respect that fact and take that into consideration when stretching. Whenever you are developing a stretching routine, always evaluate the benefits versus risk of each stretch. Not every stretch is right for everyone. Treat the selection of stretches in this book as a menu and pick only those that "feel" good to you. Two hours after stretching, you should *not* feel worse than when you started.

Listen to your body and foster body wisdom. Make your flexibility program an integrated mind-body experience. Turn your interests inward when you stretch. Reflex and relax. If your mind is uptight, it will be hard to relax your body. Some people enjoy listening to soft music while performing the stretch-and-relax portion of the program. If something hurts, stop immediately; consult your physician for unusual or continuous pain.

Be mindful of your movements. Move slowly between positions of lying down, sitting or standing—don't overestimate your body's capacity to exercise. However, don't underestimate it, either. Remember, your body is designed for movement, but let it adapt slowly and gradually.

Breathe fully while stretching. We often forget the importance that breathing has on health. Just think how women use breathing to assist in delivering a baby. Most of us take shallow breaths rather than deep full breaths. Teach yourself to breathe slowly and deeply in through your nose and exhale slowly through your lips. You will know if you are breathing correctly if your belly expands. Pattern yourself after the way a baby breathes. If you notice your ribs expanding, you are employing the wrong set of breathing muscles. Breathing fully improves the quality of a stretch. An effective method to stretch a tight muscle is to inhale first and exhale into the stretch. If you are tight in a certain muscle group, after reaching a comfortable distance, hold that position for a moment, take in a deep breath and exhale and reach a little farther. This is called the "hold/relax" method of stretching and relaxing.

Remember to stretch opposing muscle groups equally in order to keep your body balanced. Our body is designed with opposing muscles. For example, you have a muscle that brings your hand to your mouth as well as an opposing muscle that takes it in the opposite direction. So if you do a muscle activity that brings your shoulders forward, do a stretch to prevent that from happening. Stretch your tight muscles and strengthen your weak ones.

To foster your mind–body connection, try to associate your body with the targeted muscle groups identified when stretching. The chart below will assist you in knowing where you should "feel" the stretch.

Stretching Tips

The following are good rules of thumb for keeping your body safe while you strive to improve its function.

1. Warm It Up

Always increase the temperature of the muscles before stretching. Think of your muscles as taffy. Imagine trying to stretch cold taffy: it would be difficult and snap. It is the same thing for your muscles. Now imagine stretching hot taffy: it would be pliable and easy to stretch. Again your muscles respond in a similar manner. If you try to stretch a cold muscle, you are at a greater risk of injury. That is why a warm bath or light walk before you stretch is a good idea. Take time to warm up then stretch—your body will thank you later.

2. Think Functional

Stretch those joints that you need in everyday life, for example, keeping your shoulders flexible so that you can reach the

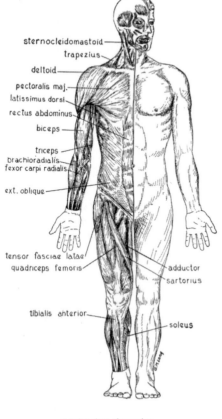

sternocleidomastoid
trapezius
deltoid
pectoralis maj.
latissimus dorsi
rectus abdominus
biceps
triceps
brachioradialis
fexor carpi radialis
ext. oblique
tensor fasciae latae
quadriceps femoris
adductor
sartorius
tibialis anterior
soleus

sternocleidomastoid
trapezius
deltoid
latissimus dorsi
triceps
brachioradialis
exten. carpi radialis
carpi ulnaris
gluteus maximus
iliotibial band
hamstrings
gastrocnemius
soleus
achilles tendon

anterior view of muscles   posterior view of muscles

Once a stretch feels completely comfortable, remember to challenge your body by holding the stretch longer or reaching further than before—but *not* to the point of pain. Ideally, it's best to work up to holding a stretch for 15 to 30 seconds. Please keep in mind that holding a stretch for 15 seconds provides a much better result than holding it for 5 seconds, and holding it for 30 seconds is better than 15 seconds. Your goal should be to be able to sustain a stretch for 30 seconds to 1 minute.

cereal box easily. You don't have to be able to tie yourself into knots, but you want to be able to perform your daily activities without undue discomfort. Stay within your comfort zone, don't ever force a move!

3. Keep It Balanced

If, for example, you do an exercise that tightens your chest muscles, spend time stretching those chest muscles.

4. Timing Is Everything

After your muscles are warmed up, try to perform each stretch 2 to 5 times and gradually try to hold each stretch 15 to 30 seconds. If 30 seconds feels okay, progress up to holding the stretch for 1 minute. No universal rule exists as to how long to hold a stretch—listen to your body!

5. Specificity of Training

Flexibility is specific to each joint. Try to stretch all the major joints of your body then focus on your particularly tight areas.

6. Do It Right

It is safer and more effective to go slow. Sustained stretches are superior to fast stretches. Bouncing, or stretching ballistically, does not increase flexibility but actually causes the stretched muscle to contract and shorten, which may induce strain or microtears of the muscle fibers.

7. "No Pain, No Gain" Is Insane

Do not stretch to the point of pain. Mild discomfort or tension is ok, but pain is not! Remember to breathe. Proper stretching should not cause pain.

8. Every Day Is Different

Many factors influence your ability to stretch. Be patient and respect these factors.

9. Individuality

Flexibility varies from day to day and from person to person; don't compete with yourself or anybody else. This is your time to savor the moment.

10. Remember the 2-Hour Rule

If you feel worse two hours after stretching, you overdid it. Next time don't do so many or reach so far.

Repetitions

This book includes active and passive stretches, both of which have their place in a comprehensive flexibility program.

Active stretches are done slowly to lubricate the joint and increase circulation in the affected area; they should be performed in your pain-free range of motion. If you have not been stretching regularly for three months, you should start out with 3–5 repetitions; if you find the first level too easy, you may want to shoot for 5–10 repetitions; if you are extremely flexible and have no joint disorders, try 10–15 repetitions.

Passive stretches are usually done when your body is warm from activity or after a bath/shower. These are static stretches held for a certain period of time. If you have not been stretching regularly for three months, hold the stretch for as long as is comfortable, working your way to 10 seconds; if you are not challenged at all by the first level, try to hold for 15–30 seconds; if you are in good shape and have no joint disorders, hold for 30–60 seconds.

Remember: For any of these stretches, listen to your body and stop if you feel discomfort or pain.

Props

The props used in this book are designed to facilitate the

stretches. However, they are not necessary. If using props is a hassle and keeps you from doing the movements, then by all means forget about them.

The **chair** provides support in balance-challenging situations. Oftentimes a wall can be used for support and balance as well.

Foam **blocks** are often used in yoga to assist in maintaining an

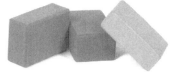

Foam blocks

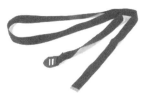

Strap with buckle

ideal position. In this book, we use blocks to serve as platforms for calf stretches and to create space in the rotator cuff exercise.

The **strap** allows you to reach the end stages of a stretch without pushing your body beyond its limits. A rope or belt can be used instead of a strap.

It's important that you are comfortable doing these stretches. When lying or kneeling on the floor, the **foam pad** provides cushioning; a **pillow** can also be used to support your neck when lying down.

Any device that facilitates your flexibility is acceptable. However, use your good judgment and always use caution when exercising.

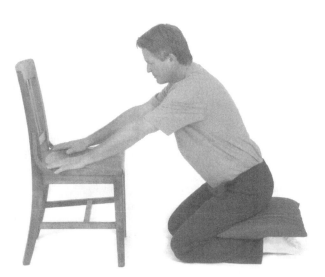

specialized
programs

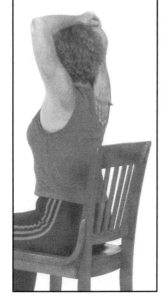

programs overview

Generally, as we get older, we lose flexibility. Many common chronic conditions cause us to "guard" or protect the joint, leading to further loss of mobility. Often, habitual overuse, either from work or play, can hasten our loss of flexibility. This section provides you with some sample stretching routines for many common chronic conditions seen in the 50-plus group. It also includes routines for recreational pursuits older adults enjoy, as well as activities done day to day.

Feel free to do some or all of the suggested stretches. Try your best to stretch daily, whether you've been very active or have been sitting for a long time. It is better to do a little bit of anything than nothing at all. Just remember to listen to your body!

Spending hours in one position (at a desk or in an airplane seat) can cause you to feel tired and stiff. The following is a simple way to stay limber:
- get up and walk around
- slowly look left and right
- squeeze your shoulder blades together
- make faces
- sit on the floor, place your legs straight out in front of you and reach forward toward your toes.

Warm Up First, Stretch After

It was not that long ago that we were instructed to stretch before engaging in sports. Even today, if you attend a high school football game, you will see the players still doing pre-game bouncing stretching, which is bad for the body whether you're 18 or 80 years of age.

It is best to warm up the muscles you plan to use with active stretches and a light jog or five-minute-long walk prior to doing any activity. Treat yourself like an expensive racehorse—no horse owner would ever allow her horse to go out on the track without being completely warmed up. So don't do anything, from shoveling snow to

golfing, without warming up your body first. Note that warming up is not the same as stretching! Do a few minutes of light activity before ever attending to your daily chores or doing your favorite sport.

The best time to stretch is after your sport/activity, when the muscles are warmed up and limber. Another good time to stretch is after a warm shower/bath. This is especially good if you have osteoarthritis.

The warm-up stretches are good to do before any activity. Start slowly and mindfully. The cool-down stretches, done after activity, will help your body release any tension or tightness you accumulated.

RECOMMENDED STRETCHES

warm-up

	PAGE	EXERCISE
	40	head tilt
	41	tennis watcher
	60	side bend
	65	seated knee to chest
	85	standing hip flexor
	87	rear calf stretch
	90	gas pedal
	94	ankle roller
	52	shoulder rolls
	47	double wood chop

cool-down

	PAGE	EXERCISE
	62	palm tree
	73	sit & reach
	65	seated knee to chest
	81	inner thighs stretch
	89	rear calf stretch with strap
	93	self ROM
	95	finger taps
	53	apple pickers
	50	elbow touches
	56	picture frame

chronic conditions

Most physical therapists and exercise physiologists agree that most of the common chronic, physical conditions can be positively influenced with sensible regular exercise. Research has shown that everything from arthritis to multiple sclerosis can benefit from a gentle stretching program.

Many of the common conditions seen in older adults make the person stiffer, which can increase pain. Flexibility training can reduce muscle injury, decrease low back pain, improve biomechanics, and reduce the stiffness of arthritis and other muscular-skeletal issues. Although all the stretching exercises in this book can be done by anyone, this section will address some common chronic conditions seen in mature adults. Nothing you do should make you feel worse; if it does, cut back a bit and re-evaluate what you are doing. Don't be afraid to consult your health professional for a selection of stretches specific to your ailments.

Arthritis
Stiffness is a common characteristic of osteoarthritis. Sensible stretching is of paramount importance in managing arthritis. Unfortunately, many people with arthritis complain of decreased flexibility, which results in a loss of range of motion.

"Use it or lose it" really pertains to arthritis: if you don't move the joint, it will become stiffer and more painful, which can impair function. This is why a water exercise program designed specifically for people with arthritis would be an excellent complement to a safe and sane stretching program approved by your health professional.

When stretching with arthritis, follow these recommendations:
- always follow medical advice
- never over-exercise
- don't mask pain with medication
- never stretch a swollen or "hot" joint
- keep movement within the pain-free range of motion

Gentle stretching can be useful, as long as you stretch the parts you're using (stretching your legs will provide little or no benefit to the shoulder region). Lastly, remember the two-hour rule: if you hurt more than two hours after exercise, back off and do less next time.

RECOMMENDED STRETCHES

arthritis

PAGE	EXERCISE
41	tennis watcher
43	turtle
65	seated knee to chest
73	sit & reach
87	rear calf stretch
92	ankle circle
90	gas pedal
100	wrist stretch seated
95	finger taps
49	rotator cuff
52	shoulder rolls

Frozen Shoulder

A frozen shoulder usually results from non-use of the shoulder because of a painful shoulder condition such as tendonitis or bursitis. If your arm is not used for a period of time, adhesions (tightness) may form on the sleeve-like structure that holds the ball and socket portion of your shoulder joint together. If the shoulder is not moved for two to three weeks, these adhesions will become very dense and strong and will result in a shoulder that cannot move freely—thus the term "frozen shoulder." If you have not been able to use your shoulder for a few months, consult a health care professional and follow a program under his or her supervision. Let pain be your guide: if stretching increases your pain, back off and follow the two-hour rule. It might be wise to warm up the joint with a heating pad prior to stretching and using ice after stretching.

Low Back Pain

Low back pain is caused by a variety of sources—weak abdominals, tight hamstrings and quadriceps, improper body mechanics, poor posture, overuse, facet and joint problems, and herniated discs. Many arm movements affect the low back; activities such as overhead reaching affect the lumbar lordosis. Back problems should be diagnosed by a health care professional. A healthy back program includes exercises that

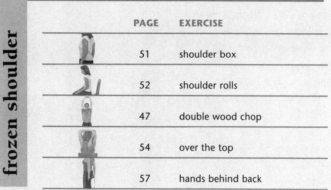

RECOMMENDED STRETCHES

frozen shoulder

	PAGE	EXERCISE
	51	shoulder box
	52	shoulder rolls
	47	double wood chop
	54	over the top
	57	hands behind back

low back pain

	PAGE	EXERCISE
	66	single knee to chest
	67	double knee to chest
	73	sit & reach
	68	double-leg stretch
	104	mad cat
	105	long body stretch
	85	standing hip flexor
	69	piriformis stretch

strengthen the abdominals and stretch the hamstrings (backs of thighs) as well as the low back muscles. For people with back problems, learning and performing good neutral spine technique is very important. See "Proper Posture" on page 12. All exercises should be done from this stance unless otherwise instructed by your health professional.

Knee Problems

Chronic knee problems can be the result of poor anatomical design. If you are bowlegged or knock-kneed, you are at a mechanical disadvantage that can set you up for injury. Foot misalignments can also contribute to knee problems. In addition, injuries from sports such as football or soccer, or even too many step aerobic classes or even badly executed stretches, can harm your knees. Your knee is an engineering marvel but can still break down if used incorrectly. Be careful to keep the knee in biomechanical alignment: your knees and toes should always point in the same direction, and you should never overbend your knees or over-straighten your legs.

Hip Problems

Designed to support the load of our body, the hips are often called the workhorse of the body. Unfortunately, some people overuse them with their jobs or in the weight room with heavy lifts. Sometimes, years of being overweight can put too much load on the joint and cause good hips to go bad. Consult your health professional for specific exercises for the hip joint. Avoid flexion past 90 degrees (allowing your knee to get too close to your chest) or crossing the midline of your body (when you swing your leg in front or behind the other leg).

Repetitive Wrist Strain

Repetitive injuries are caused from—just as they sound—doing any detailed task without taking a break. The pathology that causes the problem is complex and needs to be explained by your doctor. An interesting thing is that carpal tunnel wrist syndrome really increased when computers became popular.

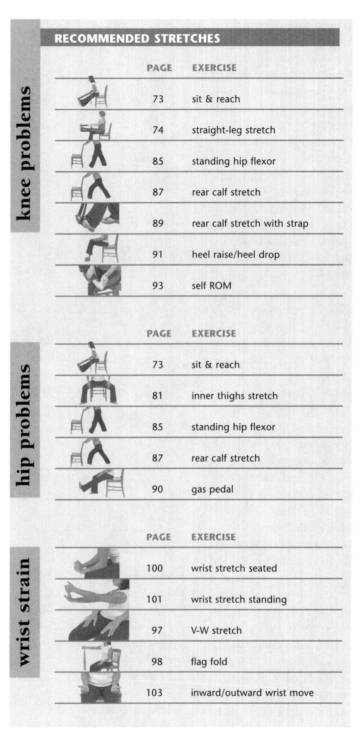

RECOMMENDED STRETCHES

knee problems

PAGE	EXERCISE
73	sit & reach
74	straight-leg stretch
85	standing hip flexor
87	rear calf stretch
89	rear calf stretch with strap
91	heel raise/heel drop
93	self ROM

hip problems

PAGE	EXERCISE
73	sit & reach
81	inner thighs stretch
85	standing hip flexor
87	rear calf stretch
90	gas pedal

wrist strain

PAGE	EXERCISE
100	wrist stretch seated
101	wrist stretch standing
97	V-W stretch
98	flag fold
103	inward/outward wrist move

recreational pursuits

This series is designed to prevent possible injuries, habilitate existing injuries, and balance out the negative results of one-sided activities such as golf and tennis.

Walking/Jogging

Jogging, running or walking is primarily a lower body activity. Start out at a slower pace than you usually do. Once you feel warmed up, stop and stretch your hips, legs, knees and ankles as well as your chest and shoulders (often your upper body becomes hunched over). After your walk, take time to stretch some more.

walking/jogging

RECOMMENDED STRETCHES

	PAGE	EXERCISE
	68	double-leg stretch
	67	double knee to chest
	81	inner thighs stretch
	85	standing hip flexor
	84	pretzel
	87	rear calf stretch
	78	side quad stretch
	88	drop-off stretch
	44	hold/relax turtle
	45	neck pull/head tilt
	90	gas pedal
	92	ankle circle
	56	picture frame

Tennis

Tennis is a fun sport, but it often takes a significant toll on the body. The knees take a pounding, the shoulders are asked to perform some difficult moves. The load placed on the spine, not to mention the cardiovascular system, is tremendous. The fact that it is mostly an asymmetrical game (meaning it is done mostly on one side of the body) sets you up for misalignments. Stretching is very important if you are a tennis player. Take a few minutes to walk around the court then gently hit the ball back and forth to lubricate the affected joints. Once you're warmed up, take a few moments to stretch before the game starts. Also stretch between sets as well as after the game.

tennis

RECOMMENDED STRETCHES

	PAGE	EXERCISE
	68	double-leg stretch
	67	double knee to chest
	69	piriformis stretch
	70	diagonal knee to chest
	82	the butterfly
	81	inner thighs stretch
	85	standing hip flexor
	87	rear calf stretch
	88	drop-off stretch
	75	V stretch
	92	ankle circle
	56	picture frame
	48	soup can pours
	58	pec stretch
	49	rotator cuff
	99	squeezer

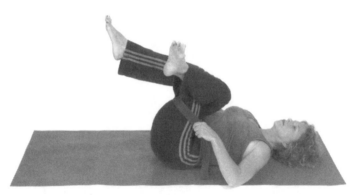

Swimming

Water exercise is gentle on the body and everybody should do it. But swimming is not as kind. Often the moves we ask the shoulders to do over time can contribute to shoulder problems and breathing to one side over and over can aggravate low back problems. A few gentle laps to warm up is always a good idea. Stretch after your laps. It would be wise to have your swim skills critiqued if you swim a lot.

swimming

RECOMMENDED STRETCHES

	PAGE	EXERCISE
	86	kneeling hip flexor
	87	rear calf stretch
	90	gas pedal
	93	self ROM
	100	wrist stretch seated
	52	shoulder rolls
	47	double wood chop
	55	choker
	54	over the top
	58	pec stretch

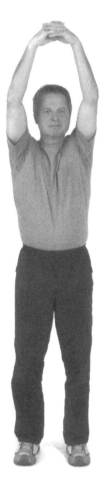

Golf

Many people say they play golf, yet I am still waiting to speak to someone who "plays" golf. Most people actually compete at golf, and often make an enjoyable pastime a stress-laden event. Golf is tough on the body, hard on the knees, hips and, especially, the low back. One problem with golf is that it is asymmetrical, meaning only one side of the body gets used over and over again. The other issue is that the worse at golf you are, the harder it is on your body due to more repetition and bad form.

Walk for a few minutes before the match starts; walk the course, if possible. Don't always pull your clubs with the same arm. Similarly, try taking an equal number of swings to the left and right to even out all the one-sided swings you'll be executing in the game. Try to stay balanced to the left as you are to the right. And finally, avoid the food and drink at the 19th hole!

golf

RECOMMENDED STRETCHES

PAGE	EXERCISE
43	turtle
40	head tilt
60	side bend
63	twister
62	palm tree
65	seated knee to chest
72	roll into a ball
67	double knee to chest
81	inner thighs stretch
86	kneeling hip flexor
87	rear calf stretch
93	self ROM
101	wrist stretch standing
102	inward/outward wrist move
96	finger spreaders
52	shoulder rolls
46	windmill
57	hands behind back
59	the zipper
50	elbow touches

Biking

Most people would assume that biking is a lower body activity. But think of your posture. Your body is rounded over the handle bars, with much of your weight resting on your wrists and hands. Start out with an easy warm-up ride. If you're very inflexible, get off the bike and stretch. Otherwise, stretch after your ride and ice sore joints if necessary. If you can, have your bike adjusted professionally to fit you.

biking

RECOMMENDED STRETCHES

PAGE	EXERCISE
66	single knee to chest
79	quad stretch
67	double knee to chest
86	kneeling hip flexor
69	piriformis stretch
85	standing hip flexor
68	double-leg stretch
76	figure 4
87	rear calf stretch
77	inverted figure 4
83	outer thigh stretch
90	gas pedal
92	ankle circle
101	wrist stretch standing
96	finger spreaders (standing)
57	hands behind back
58	pec stretch
50	elbow touches
52	shoulder rolls

Skiing

Skiing can be an explosive sport that asks you to perform hard for short spurts, stand around for awhile in line and then exert full force again. With skiing, you have to contend with the cold and high altitudes, and our fifty-plus tendons/ligament often gel up when left alone in the cold. Skiing is a total body sport, and can be hard on shoulders, knees and tendons. Always warm up and stop when you are fatigued. Listen to your body. Don't over-ski your ability or fitness level. Ski a couple of bunny slopes before you start off the day. Stretch after a warm shower.

skiing

RECOMMENDED STRETCHES

PAGE	EXERCISE
42	skyscraper
62	palm tree
60	side bend
73	sit & reach
79	quad stretch
80	kneeling quad stretch
85	standing hip flexor
87	rear calf stretch
92	ankle circle
100	wrist stretch seated
96	finger spreaders
47	double wood chop
55	choker
56	picture frame
54	over the top

Rowing, Canoeing or Kayaking

Rowing is primarily an upper body task, so pay attention to not getting overly tight through the chest region.

Perform a light walk or jog beforehand. If you tend to use only one side to stroke, try to switch sides in order to balance out your muscle use.

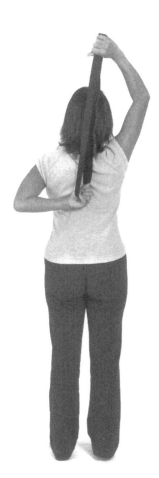

rowing, canoeing or kayaking

RECOMMENDED STRETCHES

	PAGE	EXERCISE
	63	twister
	41	tennis watcher
	40	head tilt
	64	cross-leg drop
	60	side bend
	67	double knee to chest
	69	piriformis stretch
	79	quad stretch
	85	standing hip flexor
	92	ankle circle
	95	finger taps
	52	shoulder rolls
	46	windmill
	58	pec stretch
	59	the zipper
	56	picture frame
	102	wrist stretch kneeling

Bowling

Many people don't think bowling is a sport, yet it can be very hard on the hips, knees, shoulders and back. One problem that bowling presents is that it is one-sided, and you are asked to throw a heavy ball full force. All this can lead to injuries. Practice with a few easy rolls before going full strength.

bowling

RECOMMENDED STRETCHES

	PAGE	EXERCISE
	73	sit & reach
	81	inner thighs stretch
	85	standing hip flexor
	87	rear calf stretch
	90	gas pedal
	91	heel raise/heel drop
	100	wrist stretch seated
	103	inward/outward wrist (standing)
	95	finger taps
	96	finger spreaders
	51	shoulder box
	53	apple pickers
	46	windmill
	58	pec stretch
	56	picture frame
	40	head tilt
	41	tennis watcher
	60	side bend
	65	seated knee to chest
	63	twister

daily activities

The following are some simple stretching routines for daily activities that seem innocuous enough but can cause problems when performed abruptly or for too long.

Gardening

Gardening sounds like fun to some and work to others. If you are not fit to bend, squat or lift, perhaps window box gardening may be a better option. Warm up the body before you start gardening. If it is spring planting and you have been sedentary all winter, use caution and don't overdo it.

RECOMMENDED STRETCHES		
	PAGE	EXERCISE
	41	tennis watcher
	42	skyscraper
	60	side bend
	63	twister
	85	standing hip flexor
	87	rear calf stretch
	100	wrist stretch seated
	95	finger taps
	53	apple pickers
	47	double wood chop
	104	mad cat

gardening

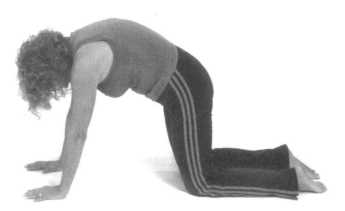

Working at a Desk or Computer

Sitting still and doing anything for a long time is not good for the body. Sitting over a computer causes you to have rounded shoulders, a protruding head and wrist problems. Get up and move around as often as possible. Stand while on the phone. Walk to deliver a message whenever possible. Set your computer to remind you to get up once every hour. Drink plenty of water/juice to make you get up often. At lunch, don't work at your desk—take a walk. Park as far away from your office as you can, and take the stairs when possible.

RECOMMENDED STRETCHES

PAGE	EXERCISE
40	head tilt
41	tennis watcher
43	turtle
60	side bend
63	twister
62	palm tree
73	sit & reach
65	seated knee to chest
81	inner thighs stretch
87	rear calf stretch
90	gas pedal
92	ankle circle
100	wrist stretch seated
95	finger taps
96	finger spreaders
51	shoulder box
52	shoulder rolls
50	elbow touches
57	hands behind back
58	pec stretch
54	over the top

Long Drive or Plane Flight

A long drive or plane flight can cause muscles to get tight. Often the upper and low back start to ache, and the shoulders and lower legs feel cramped. Sitting for a long time will not only make you inflexible but can be hazardous to your health. There is a condition called "economy class" syndrome, when people sit for a prolonged period of time; the worst-case scenario is death. Get up as often as possible, drink water, avoid alcohol and stretch regularly.

long drive or plane flight

RECOMMENDED STRETCHES

	PAGE	EXERCISE
	41	tennis watcher
	43	turtle
	40	head tilt
	85	standing hip flexor
	87	rear calf stretch
	90	gas pedal
	91	heel raise/heel drop
	100	wrist stretch seated
	95	finger taps
	96	finger spreaders
	51	shoulder box
	52	shoulder rolls

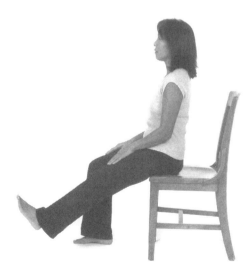

Housecleaning/Lifting

Doing housework can be strenuous physical activity and caution needs to be used because it is very easy to strain muscles. Areas of special concern should be the low back and knees. Walk around for a few minutes before doing chores and then stretch afterwards. Protect your back and ask for help when needed. Use step ladders rather than a chair to reach high places. Be careful when vacuuming or making the bed, which are hard on your low back.

housecleaning/lifting

RECOMMENDED STRETCHES

	PAGE	EXERCISE
	65	seated knee to chest
	73	sit & reach
	81	inner thighs stretch
	87	rear calf stretch
	92	ankle circle
	91	heel raise/heel drop
	95	finger taps
	99	squeezer
	52	shoulder rolls
	47	double wood chop
	46	windmill
	56	picture frame

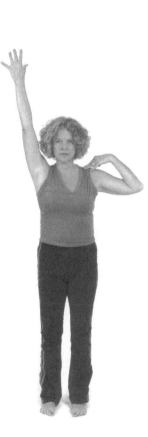

Shoveling Snow

Anyone who has ever shoveled
snow knows how tough this task
can be. How often do you pick
up the paper to read about
someone dying as a result of
shoveling snow? Shoveling is
hard on the whole body, but
especially your low back. Always
warm up first. Don't hurry or
strain—it could kill you! This
may be an activity that's better to
hire a kid to do, rather than pay
a doctor to fix your back or an
emergency room doctor to fix
your heart attack. If you feel that
your heart and breathing rate are
elevated as you're shoveling, stop
and check them. If they are high,
slow down or stop.

shoveling snow

RECOMMENDED STRETCHES

	PAGE	EXERCISE
	60	side bend
	73	sit & reach
	72	roll into a ball
	85	standing hip flexor
	91	heel raise/heel drop
	53	apple pickers
	47	double wood chop
	46	windmill
	104	mad cat

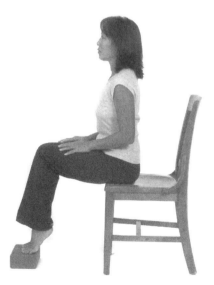

38

Bed Stretches

Many of us with chronic pain or stiffness wake up tight in the morning. Many times it is a good idea to take a few moments to make note of what is clicking and crunching. Slowly move your body through a comfortable range of motion. Use your cat or dog as a model. Animals often stretch before they jump up and play. If dogs and cats do it, why don't humans do it? Sometimes getting up and taking a warm shower and then doing some easy stretches on or in the bed is a good way to start the day.

bed stretches

RECOMMENDED STRETCHES

	PAGE	EXERCISE
	61	knee roll
	66	single knee to chest
	73	sit & reach (in bed)
	71	rock 'n' roll
	72	roll into a ball
	67	double knee to chest
	90	gas pedal
	93	self ROM
	95	finger taps
	58	pec stretch
	49	rotator cuff

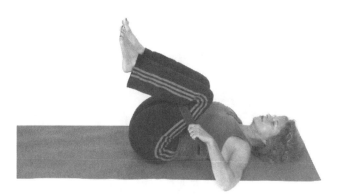

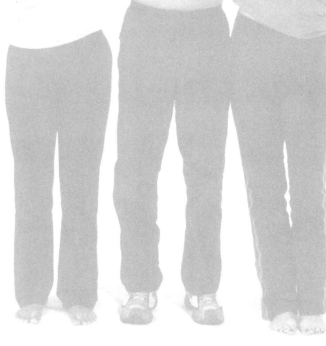

part three:
the
stretches

head tilt

starting position

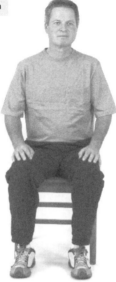

You can also try this stretch standing with proper posture.

STARTING POSITION: Sit with proper posture in a stable chair.

1 While inhaling slowly through your nose, slowly tilt your head toward your left shoulder. Keep your shoulders down and relaxed. Exhale slowly through your lips and hold this position for a moment, feeling the stretch.

2 Now inhale slowly through your nose and slowly tilt your head to your right shoulder. Exhale slowly through your lips and hold this position for a moment, feeling the stretch.

Repeat as desired.

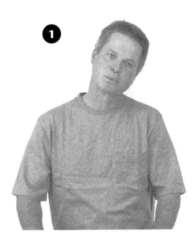

❶

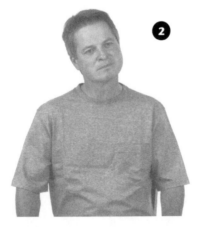

❷

starting position

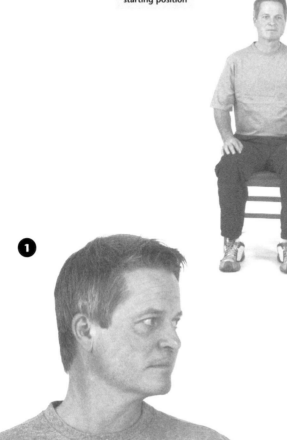

You can also try this stretch standing with proper posture.

STARTING POSITION: Sit with proper posture in a stable chair.

1 While inhaling slowly through your nose, look to your left as far as you can without feeling discomfort. Exhale slowly through your lips and hold this position for a moment, feeling the stretch.

2 Now inhale slowly through your nose and look slowly to the right. Exhale slowly through your lips and hold this position for a moment, feeling the stretch.

Repeat as desired.

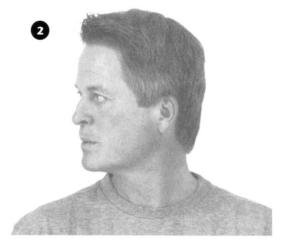

skyscraper

starting position

CAUTION: *Avoid hyperextending and hyperflexing the neck. If you have a history of neck problems, do not do this move.*

You can also try this stretch standing with proper posture.

STARTING POSITION: Sit with proper posture in a stable chair. Position your chin so that it's parallel with the floor.

1 While inhaling slowly through your nose, tilt your head just slightly to look up to the ceiling. Don't arch your neck. Hold this position for a moment, feeling the stretch.

2 Now exhale through your lips and lower your chin to your chest just slightly.

Repeat as many times as feels comfortable.

starting position

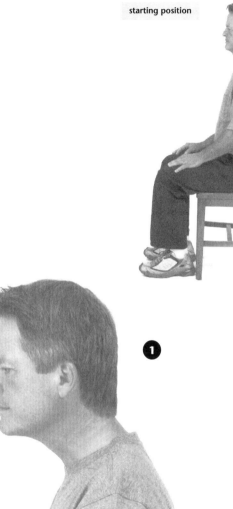

This exercise is designed to reverse the effects of "forward" head, a common result of sitting in front of a computer for hours. You can also try this stretch standing with proper posture.

STARTING POSITION: Sit with proper posture in a stable chair. Pretend you're holding an apple under your chin, or keep your chin parallel with the floor. Inhale deeply.

1 While exhaling through your lips, push your chin forward.

2 Now inhale through your nose and slowly pull your head back to the starting position. The focus of this exercise is to pull the head back.

Repeat this move as many times as feels comfortable.

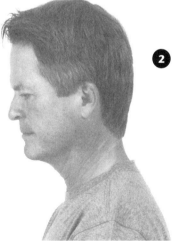

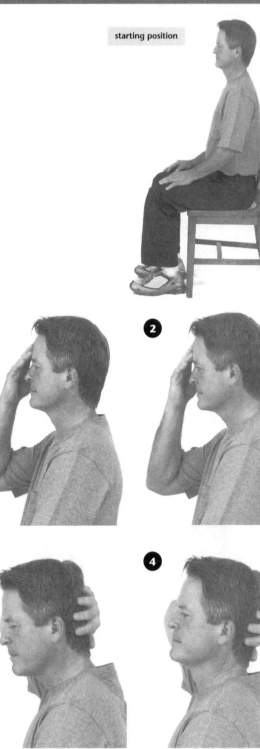

starting position

This exercise is designed to reverse the effects of "forward" head, a common result of sitting in front of a computer for hours. You can also try this stretch standing with proper posture.

STARTING POSITION: Sit with proper posture in a stable chair. Pretend you're holding an apple under your chin, or position your chin so that it's parallel with the floor.

1 Position the fingertips of your right hand on the center of your forehead. Focus on your deep breathing techniques.

2 Gently press your forehead into your fingertips. Stay mindful of your breathing and hold this position for a comfortable moment.

3 Return to starting position, then place your right hand on the back of your head.

4 Now breathe deeply in through your nose and push your skull into your hand. Place more emphasis on this phase of the exercise. Stay mindful of your breathing and hold this position for a comfortable moment.

Release and return to starting position.

MODIFICATION

Instead of using your fingertips, you can press your head into a pillow held in your hand.

If your right shoulder is tight, use your left hand, and vice versa.

starting position

CAUTION: *If you have a history of neck problems (e.g., herniated discs, arthritis of the neck), consult a health professional before performing this move.*

You can also try this stretch standing with proper posture.

STARTING POSITION: Sit with proper posture in a stable chair.

1 While inhaling deeply through your nose, slowly tilt your head to the left.

2 Once in this position, place the fingertips of your left hand on the right side of your head. While exhaling through your lips, *gently* pull your head to your left shoulder. Keep your shoulders relaxed and down. Hold this position and continue to breathe deeply in through your nose and out through your lips.

Release and return to starting position. Repeat on the other side.

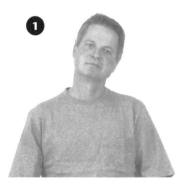

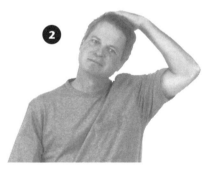

windmill

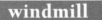

starting position

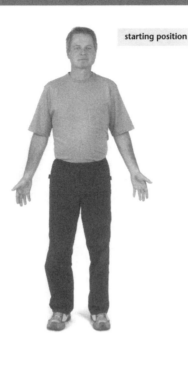

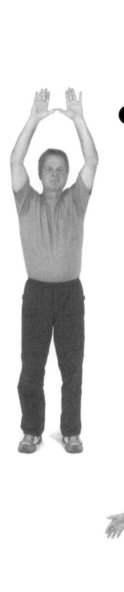

STARTING POSITION: Stand with proper posture, your arms at your sides, palms facing forward.

1 Inhale deeply through your nose and slowly raise your arms out to the side as high as is comfortable. Try to touch your thumbs.

2 Exhale and slowly lower your arms.

Repeat as desired.

MODIFICATION
This exercise can also be done one arm at a time.

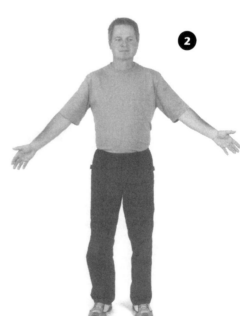

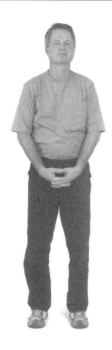

starting position

STARTING POSITION: Stand with proper posture. Position your hands in front of your body and interlace your fingers.

1 Inhale deeply through your nose and slowly raise both arms in front of you to a comfortable height. Hold 1–2 seconds.

2 Slowly lower your arms to starting position.

Repeat as desired.

1

2

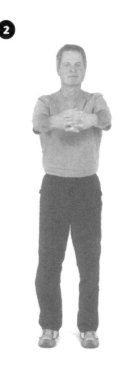

soup can pours

starting position

STARTING POSITION: Stand with proper posture, your arms at your side and your palms facing back.

1 Inhale deeply through your nose and bring both arms slightly forward as your raise them out to the sides, keeping your palm facing back. Raise your arms no higher than shoulder level.

2 Exhale as you lower your arms.

Repeat as desired.

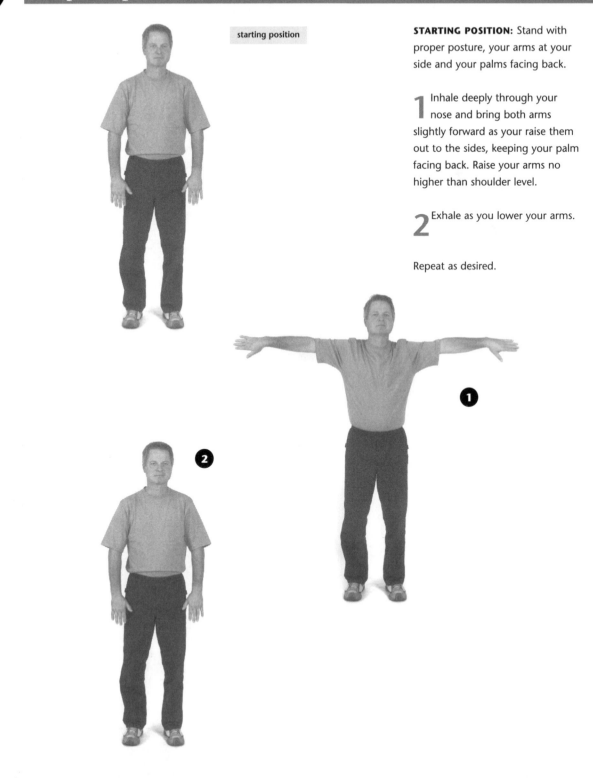

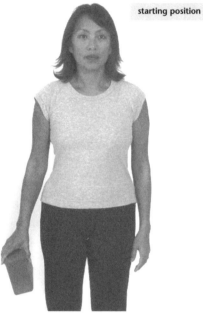

starting position

You can substitute a rolled-up towel for the block.

STARTING POSITION: Stand with proper posture with your arms at your sides. Hold a block in your right hand.

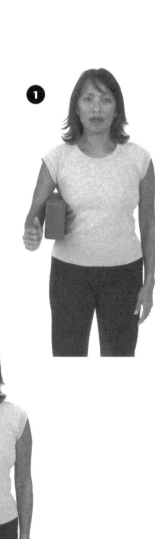

1 Squeeze the block between your right arm and your torso and bend your right elbow 90 degrees. Point your thumb up.

2 Keeping your elbow as close to your body as possible and your forearm parallel to the floor, rotate your forearm out to the side.

Rotate your forearm back in toward your body. Repeat as desired then switch sides.

VARIATION

Try this with your palm facing down or up.

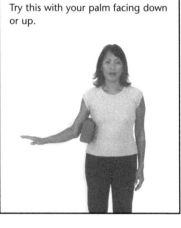

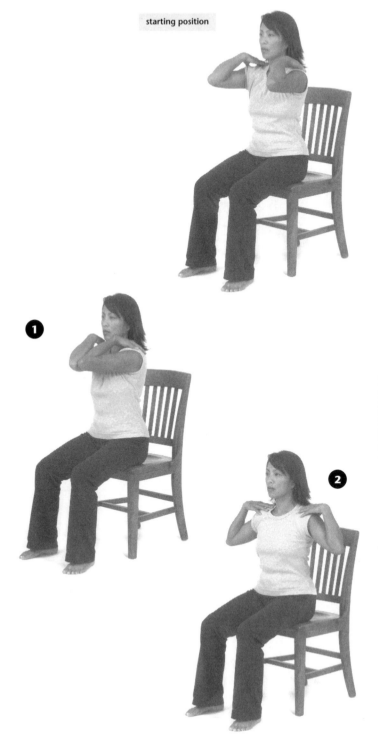

starting position

You can also try this stretch standing with proper posture.

STARTING POSITION: Sit with proper posture in a stable chair. Place your hands on your shoulders, elbows pointing forward.

1 Slowly bring your elbows together in front of your body.

2 Bring your elbows back and squeeze your shoulder blades together. Hold for a moment, focusing on opening up your chest.

Bring your elbows back to the starting position and repeat as desired.

VARIATION
Once you've done Step 2, draw circles with your elbows.

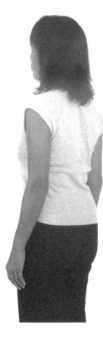

starting position

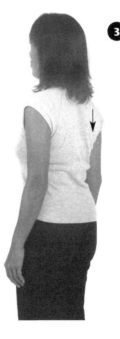

STARTING POSITION: Stand with proper posture.

1 Inhaling deeply through your nose, slowly lift up your shoulders.

2 Now pull your shoulders back and squeeze the shoulder blades together and down.

3 Exhaling through your lips, drop your shoulders and return to starting position.

Repeat as desired.

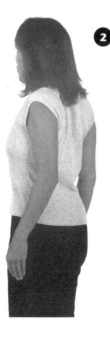

shoulder rolls

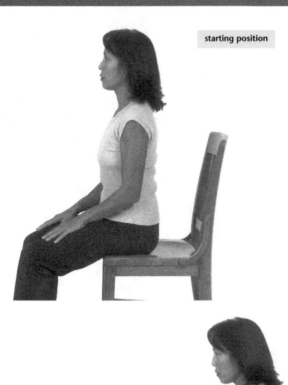

starting position

You can also try this stretch standing with proper posture.

STARTING POSITION: Sit with proper posture in a stable chair. Inhale slowly and deeply through your nose.

1 Exhaling through your nose, roll your shoulders forward, attempting to touch your shoulders together.

2 Now inhale and focus on squeezing your shoulder blades together, moving your shoulders back and opening up your chest.

Repeat as desired.

1

2

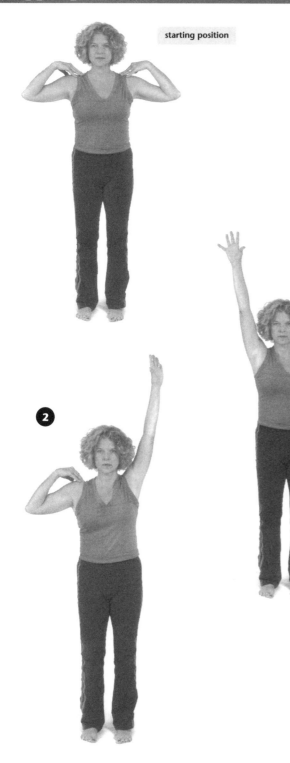

starting position

STARTING POSITION: Stand with proper posture and place your hands on your shoulders.

1 Reach your right hand as high upward as is comfortable.

2 Place the right hand back on your shoulder. Now reach up with your left hand.

Repeat as desired.

over the top

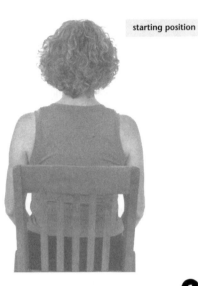

starting position

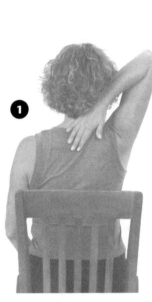

1

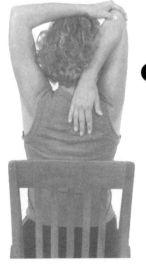

2

You can also try this stretch standing with proper posture.

STARTING POSITION: Sit with proper posture in a stable chair.

1 Raise your right arm and place your hand on your back, over your right shoulder.

2 Place your left hand on your right elbow and gently press your right arm down your back as far as feels comfortable. Hold the position for a comfortable moment.

Switch sides and repeat.

VARIATION

In Step 2, press your right arm down as you push your right elbow up into your hand. Hold this position for a comfortable moment, remembering to breathe. Then release and allow your hand to slide a little further down your back.

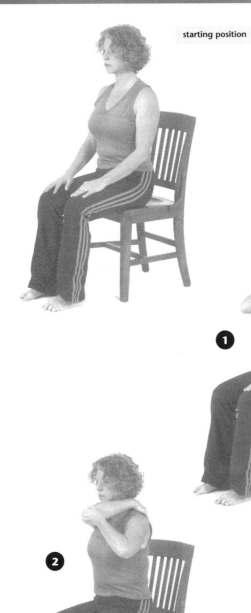

starting position

You can also try this stretch standing with proper posture.

STARTING POSITION: Sit with proper posture in a stable chair.

1 Place your right hand on your left shoulder.

2 Place your left hand on your right elbow and gently press your right elbow toward your throat. Hold for a comfortable moment.

Switch sides and repeat.

VARIATION

In Step 2, press your right elbow into your left hand. Hold for a comfortable moment, remembering to breathe. Then release to reach the right hand a little farther back.

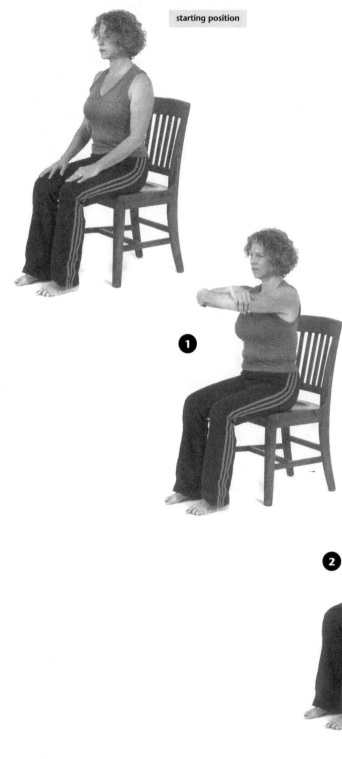

starting position

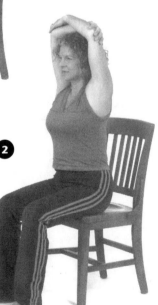

Remember not to let your low back arch. You can also try this stretch standing with proper posture.

STARTING POSITION: Sit with proper posture in a stable chair.

1 Place your right hand on your left elbow and your left hand on your right elbow.

2 Slowly lift your arms overhead, raising your arms as high as feels comfortable. Hold the position for a moment. You are now framing your face in a picture frame created by your arms—smile.

Repeat as desired.

starting position

You can also use a bar instead of a strap.

STARTING POSITION: Stand with proper posture.

1 Hold the ends of a strap in each hand behind your bottom.

2 Attempt to straighten your arms behind you. Focus on squeezing your shoulder blades together. Hold this position for as long as is comfortable.

1

2

ADVANCED

Instead of using a strap, interlock your hands behind your back.

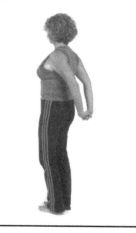

pec stretch

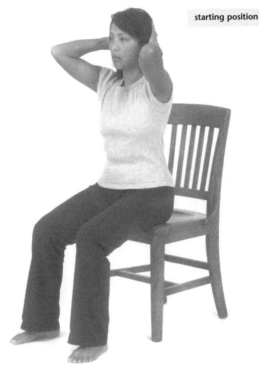

starting position

You can also try this stretch standing with proper posture.

STARTING POSITION: Sit with proper posture in a stable chair. Place your hands behind your head.

1 Gently move your elbows back and try to bring your shoulder blades together. Focus on opening up the chest and tightening the upper back muscles. Only go as far back as is comfortable and hold for a moment.

Repeat as desired.

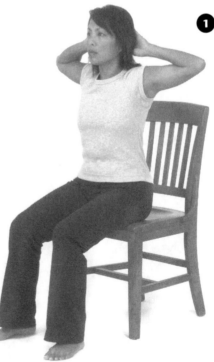

1

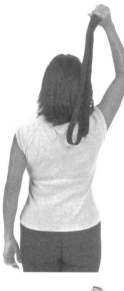

starting position

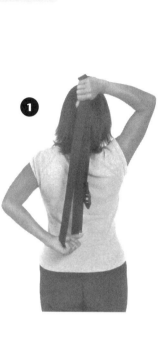

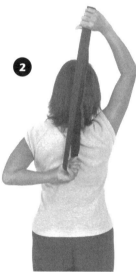

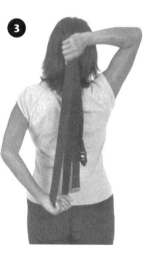

You can also try this stretch standing with proper posture.

STARTING POSITION: Stand with proper posture. Hold a strap in your right hand and raise your arm above your head.

1 Bring your right hand down behind your head and grab the dangling end of the strap with your lower hand.

2 Raise your right hand up as high as possible to lift the lower hand, staying in your pain-free zone. Hold the position for a comfortable moment.

3 Pull down with the lower hand to bring down the higher hand. Hold the position for a comfortable moment.

Switch sides and repeat.

ADVANCED

As you become more flexible, eliminate the use of the strap and try to grab your fingertips.

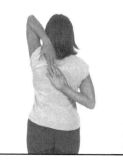

starting position

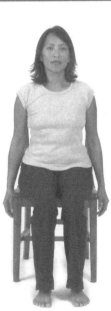

1

CAUTION: Be careful if you have low back pain.

You can also try this stretch standing with proper posture.

STARTING POSITION: Sit with proper posture in a stable chair.

1 Raise your right arm over your head to a comfortable height. Inhale deeply through your nose.

2 Now exhale through your lips and slowly and carefully lean to the left. Once you have leaned over enough to feel a gentle stretch along the right side of your body, hold this position for a comfortable moment.

Switch sides and repeat.

2

MODIFICATIONS

If your shoulder is stiff, place your hand on top of your head.

If raising your arm at all is very painful, just leave your arm alongside your body.

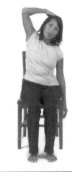

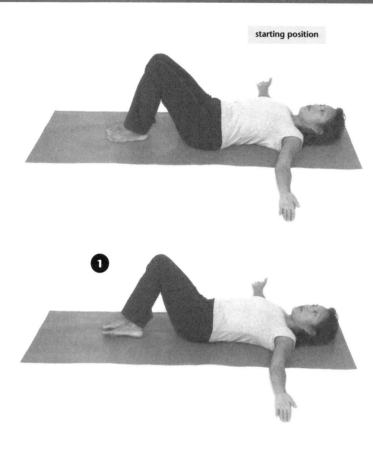

starting position

1

2

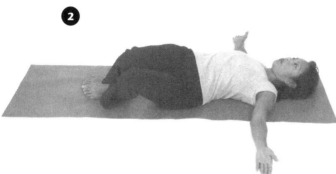

CAUTION: If you have low back problems, avoid this move.

STARTING POSITION: Lie on a mat with your knees bent and your feet flat on the floor. Place your arms straight out to your side in a "T" position.

1 While inhaling through your nose, allow your knees to drop gently to the right without discomfort. Exhale and hold this position for a comfortable moment.

2 Inhale and bring your knees back to center, then gently drop them to your left. Exhale and hold this position for a comfortable moment.

palm tree

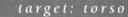
starting position

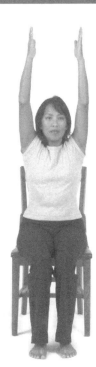

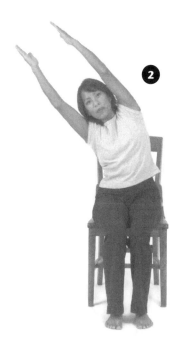

CAUTION: *If you have poor balance or low back problems, avoid this move.*

You can also try this stretch standing with proper posture.

STARTING POSITION: Sit with proper posture in a stable chair. Raise your hands overhead with your arms as straight as feels comfortable. Inhale deeply through your nose

1 While exhaling through your lips, slowly lean to your left. Hold the position for a comfortable moment, feeling the stretch along the right side of your body.

2 Now inhale fully and deeply through your nose and lean to your right. Hold this position for a comfortable moment.

ADVANCED
Try pressing your hands together as you do the side bends.

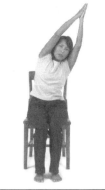

starting position

CAUTION: *Be careful if you have low back problems.*

You can also try this stretch standing with proper posture.

STARTING POSITION: Sit with proper posture in a stable chair. Cross your arms in front of your chest and inhale slowly and deeply through your nose.

1 While exhaling through your lips, slowly twist to your left. Hold the position for a comfortable moment and feel the stretch in your torso.

2 Inhale and return to the starting position before exhaling and twisting to your right. Hold the position for a comfortable moment and feel the stretch in your torso.

cross-leg drop

target: torso, piriformis

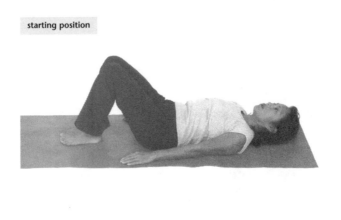

CAUTION: *Be careful if you have low back problems.*

STARTING POSITION: Lie on a mat with your knees bent and your feet flat on the floor.

1 While focusing on your breathing, place your right knee on top of your left knee.

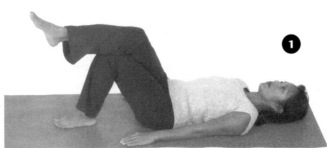

2 Slowly allow your right knee to gently fall toward the left side. Stop when you feel tightness. Hold this position for a comfortable moment. The stretch should be felt near the rear pocket area of the right leg. Focus on the stretch, not on how close you can bring the knees to the floor.

Switch sides and repeat.

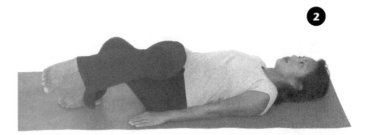

starting position

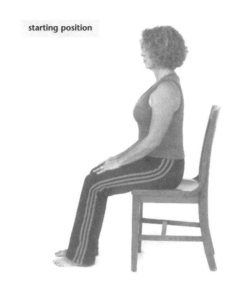

STARTING POSITION: Sit with proper posture in a stable chair and place your feet on the floor.

1 Clasp both hands beneath your left leg.

2 Bring your left knee toward your chest. Hold this position for a comfortable moment, feeling the stretch in the gluteal region.

Release the knee, switch sides and repeat.

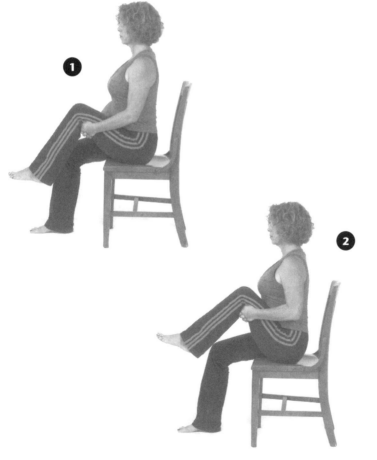

single knee to chest *target: low back, gluteus maximus*

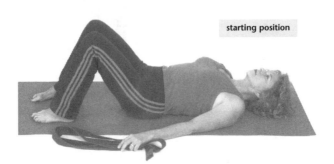

starting position

STARTING POSITION: Lie on a mat and, if needed, place a pillow under your head. Bend your knees and place both feet flat on the floor.

1 Loop a strap behind the back of your right leg and hold an end of the strap in each hand.

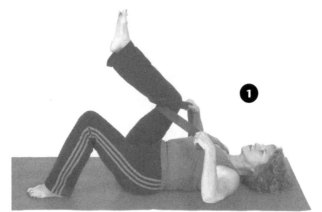

2 Gently pull the straps to bring the knee toward your chest. Hold this stretch for a comfortable moment.

Release the knee, switch sides and repeat.

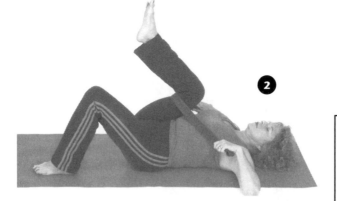

INTERMEDIATE
This can also be done using just the hands to bring in the knee.

ADVANCED
Extend one leg straight on the floor and bring one knee to your chest.

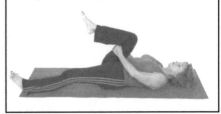

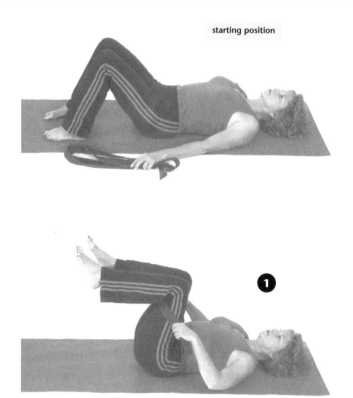

starting position

STARTING POSITION: Lie on a mat and, if needed, place a pillow under your head. Bend your knees and place both feet flat on the floor.

1 Loop a strap behind the backs of both legs and hold an end of the strap in each hand.

2 Gently pull the straps to bring your knees to your chest. Hold this position for a comfortable moment, feeling the stretch in your bottom and low back.

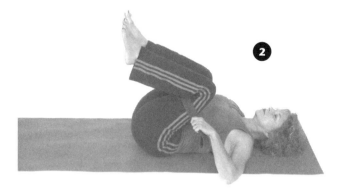

ADVANCED

Use just your hands to draw in your knees.

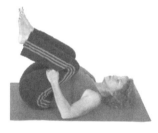

double-leg stretch

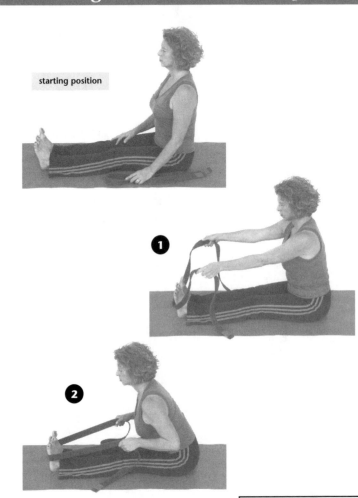

starting position

STARTING POSITION: Sit on a mat, with both legs straight out in front of you and your toes pointing up.

1 Loop a strap around your feet and hold an end of the strap in each hand.

2 Gently pull yourself forward, keeping your back straight while you reach as far forward as is comfortable. Hold for as long as is comfortable, feeling the stretch in your low back and the backs of your legs. Focus on keeping the legs straight.

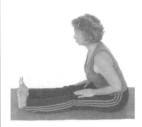

MODIFICATIONS

If you don't have a strap, you can gently press your thighs to the floor, your palms down on your thighs.

If you have a partner, have him/ her gently push you forward.

ADVANCED

Interlace your fingers and reach forward, keeping your arms parallel to the floor.

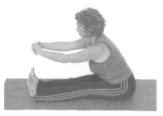

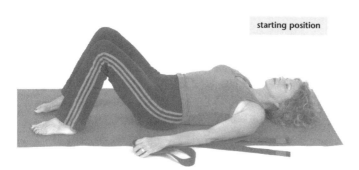

starting position

The piriformis muscle is a deep-lying muscle in the gluteal region, through which the sciatic nerve passes. When the piriformis is too tight, it can cramp the sciatic nerve, causing the symptoms of sciatica.

STARTING POSITION: Lie on a mat with your knees bent and your feet flat on the floor.

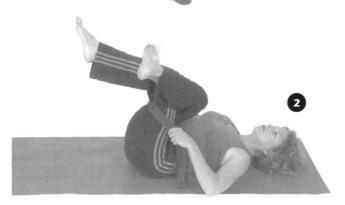

1 Cross your right knee on top of your left knee.

2 Loop a strap around both legs and pull your knees in toward your chest. Stop when tension occurs. Hold this position for a comfortable moment, focusing on the sensation of the stretch.

Switch sides and repeat.

ADVANCED

Use only your hands to pull your knees in.

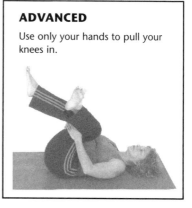

diagonal knee to chest
target: gluteus maximus, torso

starting position

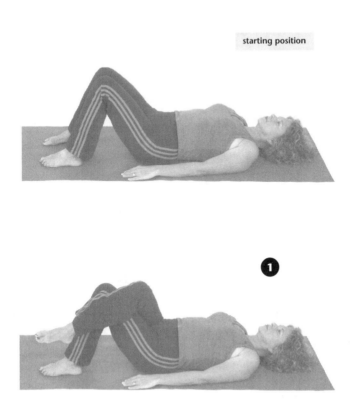

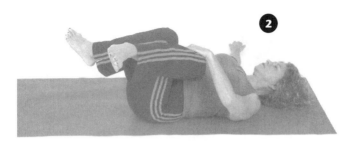

CAUTION: *Avoid this stretch if you have hip problems.*

STARTING POSITION: Lie on a mat with your knees bent and your feet flat on the floor.

1 Place your right knee on top of your left knee.

2 Draw your knees in toward your chest and pull your right knee toward your left shoulder using your left hand. Hold for a comfortable moment, focusing on the sensation of the stretch, not on how close your knee comes to your shoulder.

Switch sides and repeat.

Modification: You can also use a strap to draw in your knees.

MODIFICATION
You can also use a strap to draw in your knees.

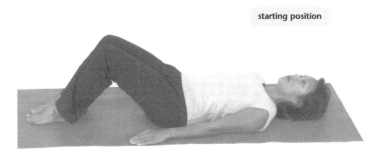

starting position

STARTING POSITION: Lie on a mat and slowly bring both knees toward your chest.

1 Gently reach around both legs and allow your shoulders to lift off the mat.

2 While inhaling deeply through your nose and exhaling through your lips, slowly rock left and right, enjoying the relaxing feeling.

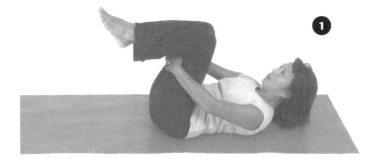

1

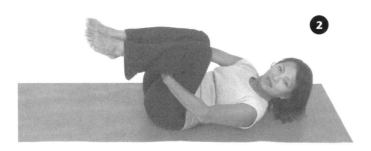

2

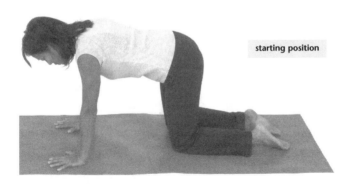

starting position

CAUTION: Do not do this stretch if you have knee problems.

STARTING POSITION: Place your hands and knees on the floor. Inhale through your nose.

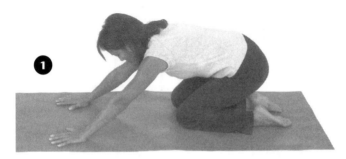

1 While exhaling deeply through your mouth, slowly allow your bottom to drop toward your heels. If you feel discomfort, you may place a pillow between your heels and bottom.

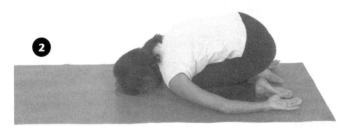

2 Place your forehead on the floor or a pillow and position your arms alongside your body. Hold this position for a comfortable moment, enjoying the sensation of the stretch up and down your back.

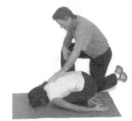

VARIATION

If you can find a friend to rub up and down your back while doing this stretch, it will enhance the stretch.

ADVANCED

Stretch your arms out straight in front of you.

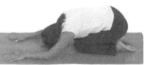

starting position

Be careful not to tip the chair over.

STARTING POSITION: Sit at the edge of a stable chair. Loop a strap around the ball of your left foot and hold an end of the strap in each hand.

1 Extend your legs straight out in front of you and place your heels on the floor with your toes pointing up 90 degrees.

2 Stack your left heel on top of your right foot, keeping your legs as straight as possible. Inhale deeply through your nose.

3 Now exhale through your lips and gently pull yourself forward by leading with your chest rather than rounding your back.

Switch sides and repeat.

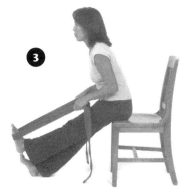

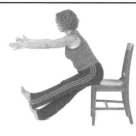

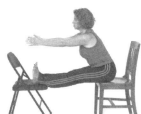

INTERMEDIATE
Instead of using the strap, you can extend your arms forward and gently reach forward with your fingertips.

ADVANCED
Place both heels on a chair in front of you.

straight-leg stretch

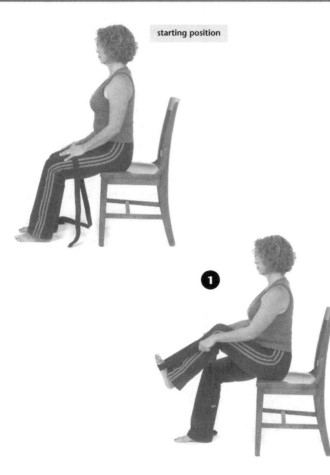

starting position

STARTING POSITION: Sit at the edge of a stable chair and place both feet flat on the floor.

1 Position a strap around the sole of the left foot and hold an end of the strap in each hand.

2 Inhale deeply through your nose and straighten your left leg. Now exhale through your lips and attempt to straighten your left leg as far as is comfortable. Hold this position for a comfortable moment.

Switch sides and repeat.

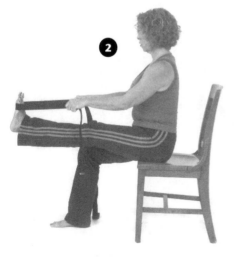

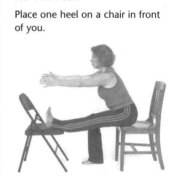

ADVANCED

Place one heel on a chair in front of you.

starting position

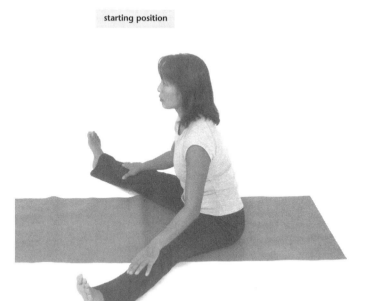

STARTING POSITION: Sit on a mat with both legs extended into a V position. Inhale deeply.

1 While keeping your head and torso tall, exhale and allow yourself to fall forward until you feel a comfortable stretch in the hamstrings and inner thighs. Be sure not to round your back. Hold this stretch for a comfortable moment, focusing on the sensation of the stretch, not on going as far as possible. Inhale through your nose and return to the starting position.

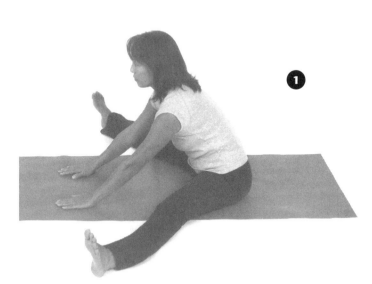

1

figure 4

starting position

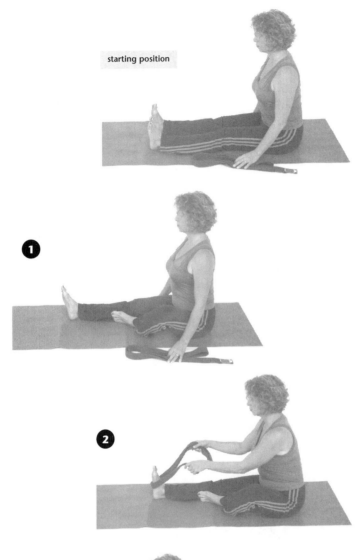

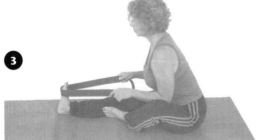

CAUTION: *Avoid this move if you have knee problems.*

STARTING POSITION: Sit on a mat with both legs extended straight out in front of you. Keep your torso as tall as possible.

1 Place your left foot against your right knee.

2 Loop a strap around the sole of your right foot and hold on to the ends of the strap. Inhale deeply through your nose.

3 While keeping your head and torso tall, pull yourself forward until you feel a comfortable stretch in the backs of your legs. Hold this stretch for a comfortable moment, focusing on the sensation of the stretch, not on going as far as possible. The goal is to hold the stretch for 60 seconds. Exhale through your lips and return to the starting position.

Switch sides and repeat.

inverted figure 4

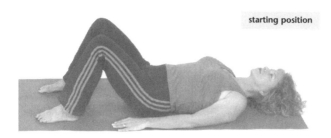

starting position

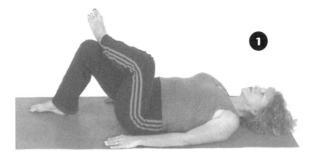

1

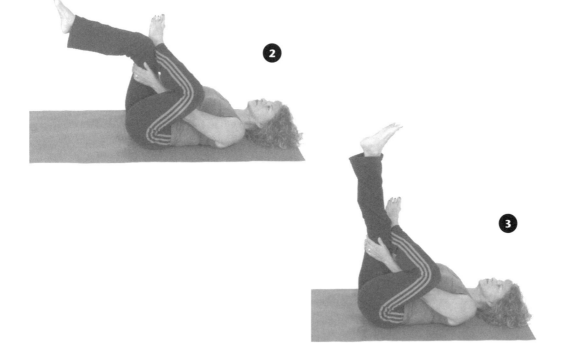

2

3

STARTING POSITION: Lie on a mat with your knees bent and your feet flat on the floor.

1 Place your left ankle on top of your right knee. Inhale deeply through your nose.

2 Wrap both hands around your right leg and bring your knee and ankle to your chest while exhaling.

3 Now straighten your right leg toward the ceiling as much as is comfortable. Focus on inhaling and exhaling fully and hold this stretch for a comfortable moment.

Switch sides and repeat.

side quad stretch

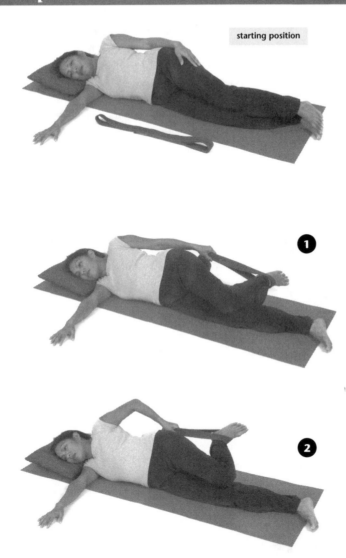

starting position

CAUTION: STOP if you notice undue compression in your knee or experience any low back discomfort. If you feel a cramp coming on, do a hamstrings stretch.

STARTING POSITION: Lie on the right side of your body on a mat. Keep your body in proper alignment: your left hip should be stacked on top of your right hip, your left knee on top of your right, your left shoulder on top of your right. Extend your bottom arm for balance.

1 Loop a strap around your left ankle.

2 Gently bring the foot back, pulling your heel toward your bottom. Hold this stretch for a comfortable moment.

Switch sides and repeat.

ADVANCED

You can try this without the strap by grasping the top of your foot.

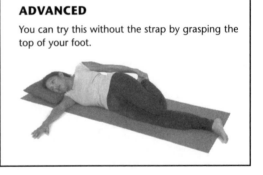

starting position

CAUTION: *Avoid this exercise if you have poor balance. STOP if you notice undue compression in your knee or experience any low back discomfort. If you feel a cramp coming on, do a hamstrings stretch.*

STARTING POSITION: Stand with proper posture facing a chair.

1 Loop a strap around your right ankle and bring your right heel toward your bottom. Keep both knees as close together as possible.

2 Gently pull your heel closer to your bottom, using the back of a chair for balance if necessary. Hold this stretch for a comfortable moment.

Switch sides and repeat.

❶

❷

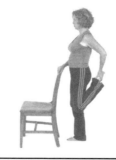

INTERMEDIATE	**ADVANCED**
Try this without the strap by grabbing your foot with your hand.	Try this without the chair, raising your free arm toward the ceiling.

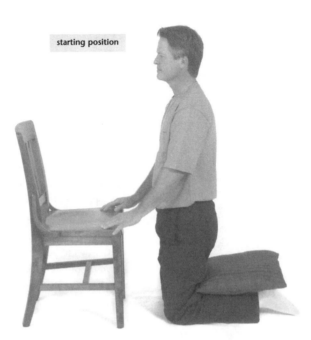

starting position

CAUTION: Avoid this move if you have knee problems.

You may want to kneel on a pad or mat to protect your knees.

STARTING POSITION: Kneel in front of a chair. Place a pillow between your heels and your bottom and place your hands on the chair.

1 Keeping both hands on the chair, slowly allow your bottom to drop toward your heels. Stop when you feel tension. Hold this stretch for a comfortable moment.

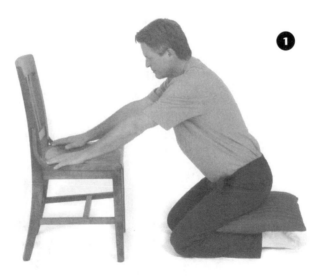

1

MODIFICATION
To increase the intensity of the stretch, use a flatter pillow or eliminate the pillow altogether.

starting position

STARTING POSITION: Sit at the edge of a stable chair and place both feet flat on the floor.

1 Spread your legs apart and point your knees and toes out to the side 45 degrees.

2 Place your hands on the insides of your thighs and gently push your legs a little wider. Hold this stretch for a comfortable moment.

Repeat as desired.

1

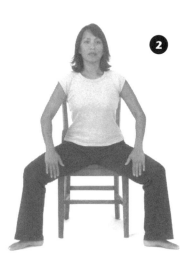

2

the butterfly

starting position

STARTING POSITION: Sit on a mat with your knees bent and your feet flat on the floor. Place the soles of your feet together and gently allow your knees to drop to the floor.

1 Loop a strap around your feet and gently pull yourself forward, not down. Hold this stretch for a comfortable moment.

Repeat as desired.

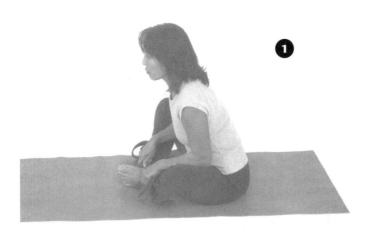

❶

ADVANCED

Place your hands on your ankles and pull yourself forward.

starting position

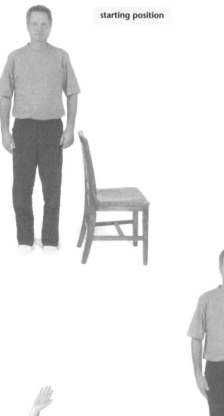

CAUTION: *If you've been advised by your doctor or therapist not to cross your legs, do not do this exercise.*

STARTING POSITION: Stand with proper posture next to a chair on your left side.

1 Cross your right leg in front of your left leg.

2 Raise your right arm up overhead and lean to the left, gently pressing your right hip outward to the right. Use the chair for balance. Hold this stretch for a comfortable moment.

Switch sides and repeat.

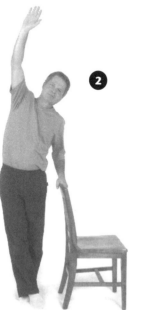

1

2

VARIATION

If your shoulders are tight, just place your hand on your hips.

ADVANCED

If balance is not an issue, try this without the chair.

pretzel

target: iliotibial band

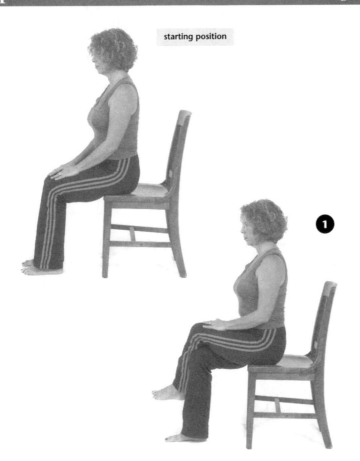

starting position

STARTING POSITION: Sit at the edge of a stable chair.

1 Cross your left knee over your right.

2 Reach both hands around the top of the left knee. Gently twist to the left while pulling the knee toward the midline of your body. Hold this stretch for a comfortable moment.

Switch sides and repeat.

❶

❷

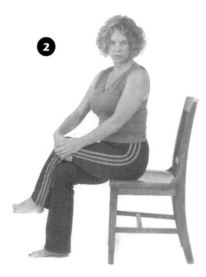

ADVANCED

This exercise can also be done sitting on the floor with your legs straight out in front of you. Bend your left knee and place your left foot on the outside of your right leg, as close to the right knee as possible. Then gently twist to the left as you look right.

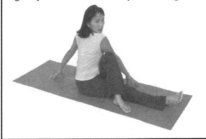

starting position

STARTING POSITION: Stand behind a chair and place your hands on the back of the chair.

1 Slide your right leg back a comfortable distance. Keeping your rear heel down, gently tuck your tailbone under and press your hips forward. Hold this stretch for a comfortable moment, focusing on feeling the stretch in the upper leg/hip region rather than in the calf area.

Switch sides and repeat.

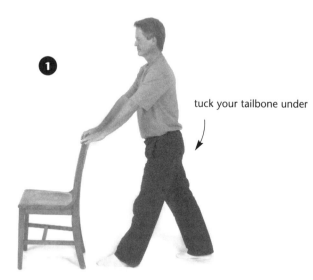

1

tuck your tailbone under

starting position

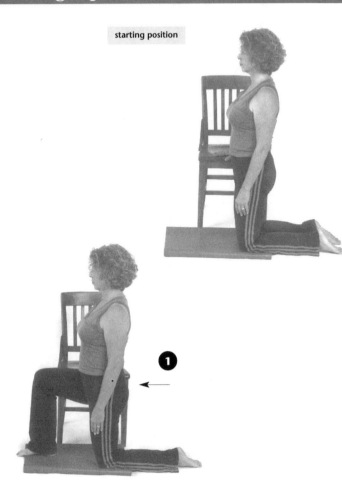

1

CAUTION: Avoid this stretch if you have poor balance and/or bad knees.

STARTING POSITION: Kneel on a mat with a chair on your right side.

1 Move your right knee forward so that you can place your right foot flat on the floor. Maintain an erect position, pulling in your chin, squeezing your shoulder blades together, and pulling in your belly button and contracting your gluteals. Slowly press your hips forward until you feel a comfortable stretch in front of your kneeling leg. Hold this stretch for a comfortable moment.

Switch sides and repeat.

INTERMEDIATE

Slide your left knee back and press up onto the ball of your foot.

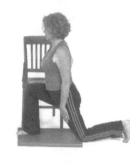

ADVANCED

You can rise onto the ball of your rear foot to lift your knee off the floor and intensify the stretch.

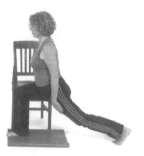

starting position

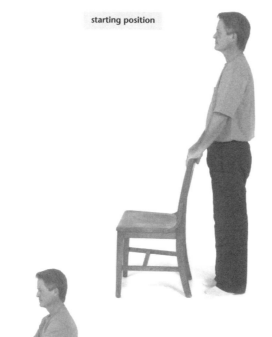

STARTING POSITION: Stand behind a chair, placing both hands on the back of the chair.

1 Keeping the heel down, slide your right leg as far back as you can.

2 Bend your left knee until the desired stretch is felt in the calf area. Hold this stretch for a comfortable moment.

Switch sides and repeat.

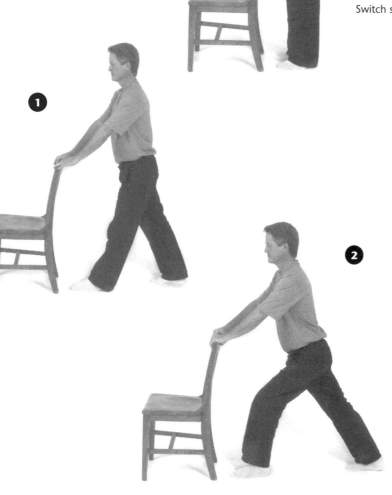

❶

❷

starting position

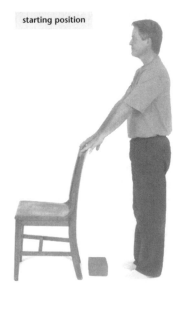

CAUTION: Only do this exercise if you're fairly flexible. Do not force anything, do not do this move if you have a history of Achilles' heel injury, and do not do if you're unsure of your balance.

STARTING POSITION: Stand behind a chair, using the back for support.

1 Place your right foot on a block.

2 Gently and slowly lower your right heel until the desired stretch is felt in the calf area. Hold this stretch for a comfortable moment, using the chair for balance if necessary.

Switch sides and repeat.

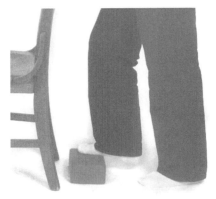

❶

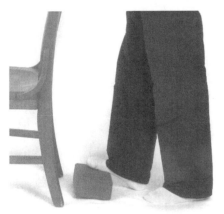

❷

starting position

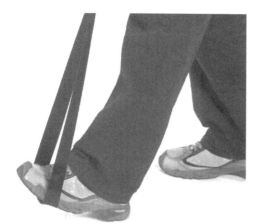

STARTING POSITION: Stand with proper posture, holding a strap in your left hand.

1 Step your left foot forward and loop the strap around the ball of the foot.

2 Keeping your heel on the floor, gently pull your toes up until you feel the desired stretch in your calf. Hold for a comfortable moment.

Switch sides and repeat.

1

2

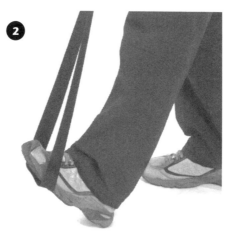

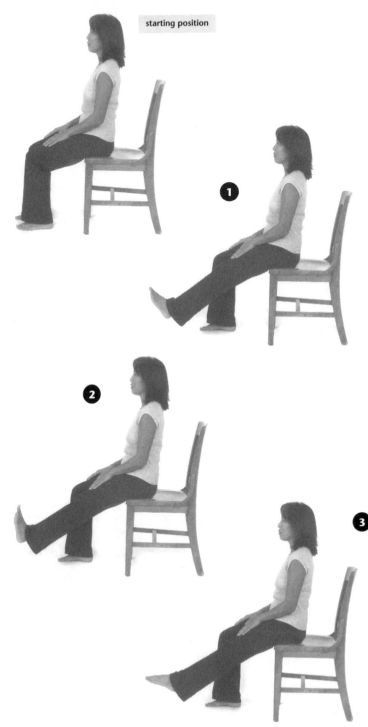

starting position

1

2

3

CAUTION: *Do not force your toes in either direction. Be aware that your calf may cramp when extending your toes.*

Be careful not to tip the chair over.

STARTING POSITION: Sit at the edge of a stable chair.

1 Extend your left leg straight out in front of you and lift it off the ground.

2 Point your toes up and hold for several seconds.

3 Extend your toes away from you and hold for several seconds.

Repeat a comfortable number of times then switch sides.

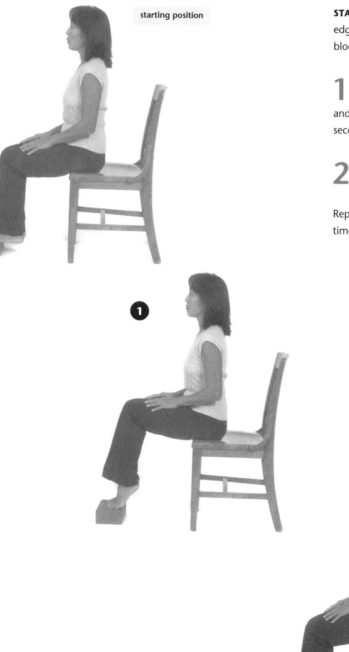

starting position

STARTING POSITION: Sit at the edge of a stable chair and place a block under the balls of your feet.

1 Keeping the balls of your feet on the block, raise your heels and hold the stretch for several seconds.

2 Drop your heels and hold the stretch for several seconds.

Repeat a comfortable number of times.

ankle circle

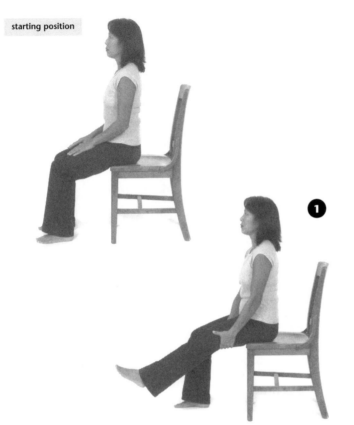

starting position

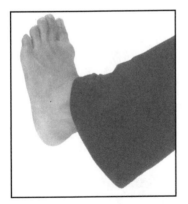

STARTING POSITION: Sit at the edge of a stable chair.

1 Extend your left leg straight out in front of you and lift it off the ground.

2 Keeping your leg stationary (using your hands for support, if necessary), point your toes and draw several circles with your foot in both directions.

Switch sides and repeat.

VARIATION

Ankle Writing: Point your toes and write your address and phone number with your foot. Switch sides and repeat.

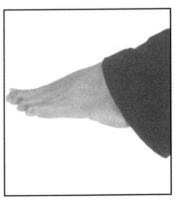

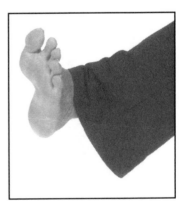

starting position

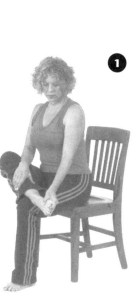

1

STARTING POSITION: Sit at the edge of a stable chair.

1 Cross your right ankle on top of your left knee and gently grasp your right foot with your left hand.

2 Slowly use your hand to gently move your foot in comfortable circles as well as forward and backward.

Switch sides and repeat.

2

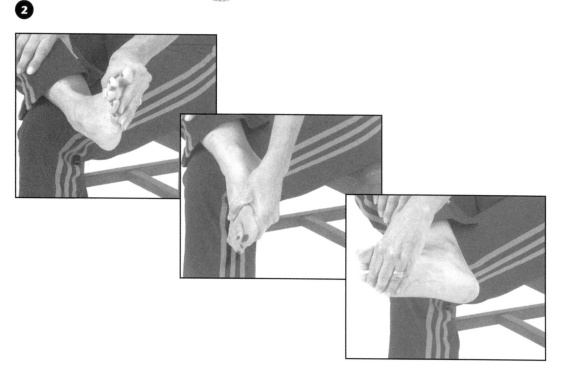

ankle roller

starting position

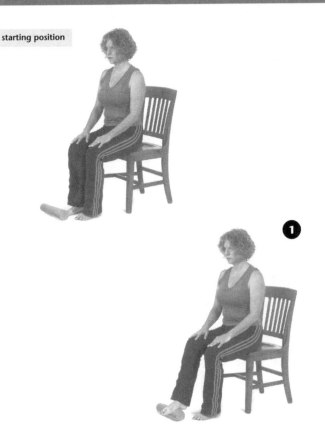

If you do not have a rolling pin, you can also use a frozen orange juice container (good for icing sore feet) or a can of soup.

STARTING POSITION: Sit at the edge of a stable chair and place both feet on the floor, directly below your knees.

1 Place a rolling pin under the arch of your right foot.

2 Slowly move your foot back and forth over the roller.

Switch sides and repeat.

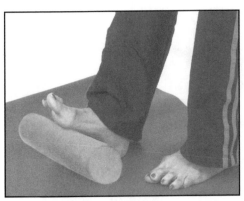
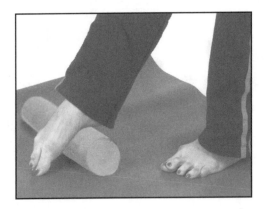

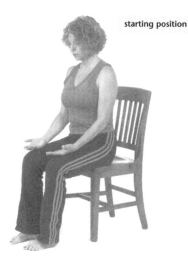

starting position

STARTING POSITION: Sit at the edge of a stable chair. Rest your hands on your thighs with your palms turned up.

1 Touch your little finger to your thumb then progress through each finger until you reach your index finger.

2 Now turn your palms down and repeat the exercise.

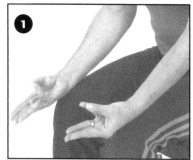

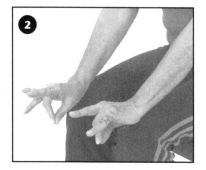

VARIATION

Finger Base Tap: Touch the thumb to the base of your little finger, then progress through each finger until you reach the index finger. Now turn your palms down and repeat the exercise.

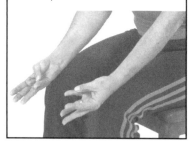

finger spreaders

starting position

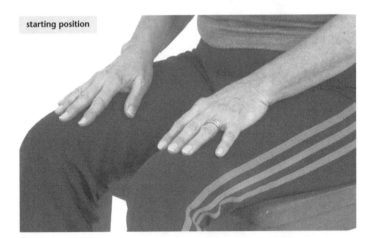

STARTING POSITION: Sit with proper posture in a stable chair. Rest your hands on your thighs with your palms down.

1 Pinch your fingers and thumb together.

2 Now separate all fingers and thumb as far apart as possible.

Turn your palms up and repeat steps 1 and 2.

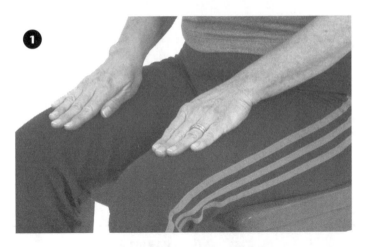

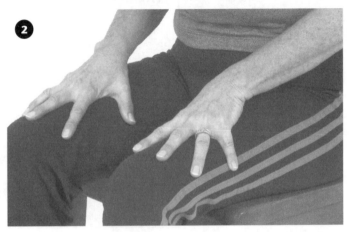

starting position

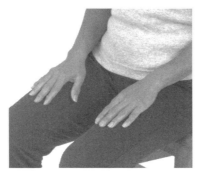

STARTING POSITION: Sit with proper posture in a stable chair. Rest your hands on your thighs with your palms down. Squeeze all your fingers together.

1 Separate one finger at a time, starting with the little finger, then the ring finger, until you've separated all your fingers. Squeeze your fingers together and repeat the exercise.

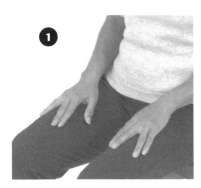

1

ADVANCED

Increase the challenge by holding your arms straight out in front of you. Instead of just separating your fingers, try to make a V and W. *To make a V:* Spread your little finger and ring finger away from your index finger and middle finger. *To make a W:* Put your ring finger and middle finger together and separate the little finger and index finger from the group.

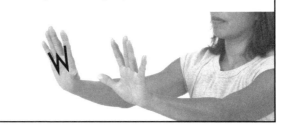

flag fold

starting position

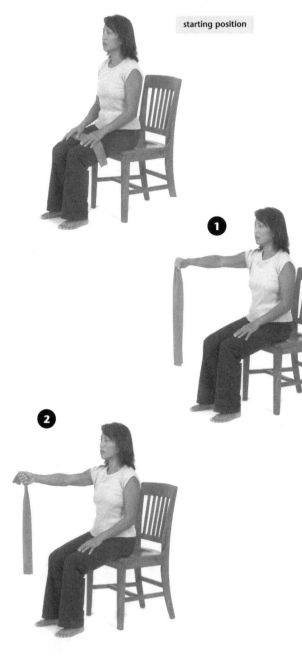

STARTING POSITION: Sit with proper posture in a stable chair.

1 Hold the end of a scarf in your right hand and extend the right arm straight out in front of you, palm down.

2 Turn your palm up and grab more scarf in your hand.

3 Turn your palm down and grab more scarf, balling up the scarf in your hand as you go. Continue until you've grabbed as much scarf as you can, then squeeze tightly several times.

Switch hands and repeat.

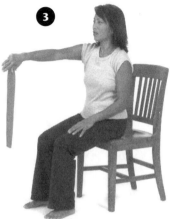

starting position

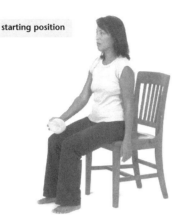

STARTING POSITION: Sit with proper posture in a stable chair.

1 Hold a small, soft, squeezable object in your right hand and extend that arm straight out in front of you. Keep your left arm by your side.

2 Slowly squeeze the object and hold for 1–2 seconds.

Repeat until the hand has done a comfortable number. Switch hands and repeat.

MODIFICATION
You can also try doing this with an object in both hands.

VARIATION
Try this on something more difficult to squeeze, like a tennis ball.

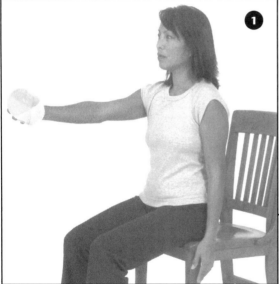

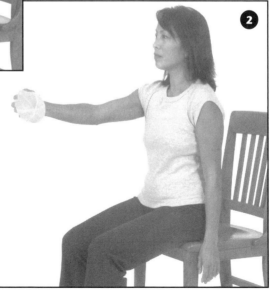

wrist stretch seated

starting position

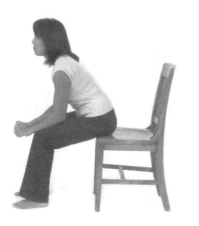

STARTING POSITION: Sit in a stable chair. Rest your forearms on your thighs so that your wrists hang off. Your hands are in a loose fist.

1 Slowly lift your knuckles toward the ceiling and hold 1–2 seconds.

2 Slowly lower your knuckles toward the floor and hold 1–2 seconds.

Repeat as feels comfortable.

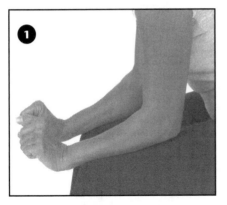

ADVANCED

After you lift your knuckles upward in Step 1, extend your fingertips, then make a fist, lower your knuckles, and extend your fingers downward.

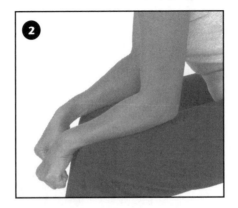

starting position

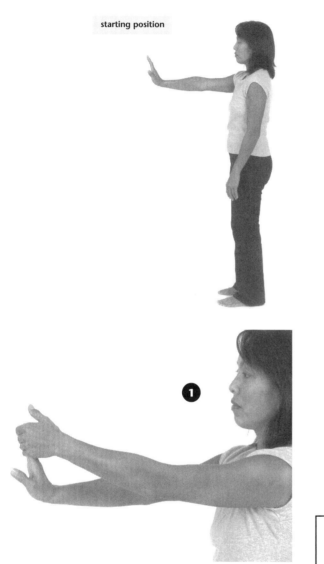

STARTING POSITION: Stand with proper posture. Extend your right arm in front of you to shoulder height, with your palm facing forward and fingers pointing toward the ceiling.

1 Gently pull your fingers back with your left hand until a desired stretch is felt under your wrist. Hold the stretch for several seconds.

Repeat as desired then switch sides.

ADVANCED

Try doing the exercise with the fingertips pointing down.

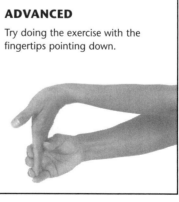

wrist stretch kneeling

This is a very advanced exercise.

STARTING POSITION: Kneel on a mat on the floor.

1 Slowly place your fingers on the floor so that your fingers are pointing toward you.

2 Slowly lower your palms to the floor without discomfort in your wrists. Be sure to keep your elbows soft. Hold the stretch for a comfortable moment.

starting position

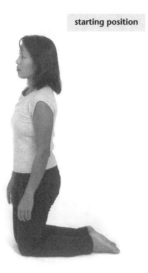

1

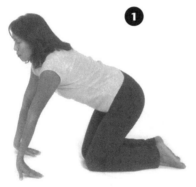

2

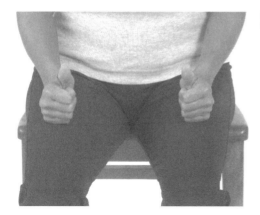

starting position

STARTING POSITION: Sit with proper posture in a stable chair. Rest your fists on your thighs with your thumbs pointing up toward the ceiling.

1 Slowly turn your fists so that your thumbs point inward.

2 Slowly turn your fists so that your thumbs point outward.

Repeat as desired.

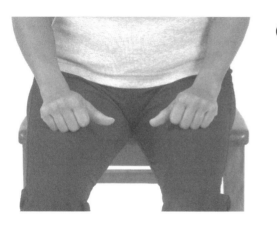

1

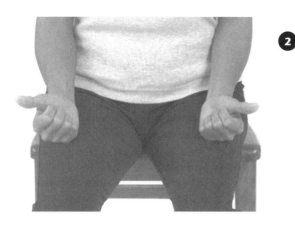

2

mad cat

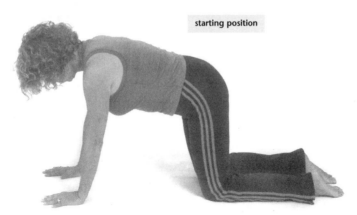

starting position

STARTING POSITION: Rest on your hands and knees.

1 Draw your belly button in, causing your back to round. Inhale deeply.

2 Now exhale and slowly relax your body to the starting position.

Repeat as desired.

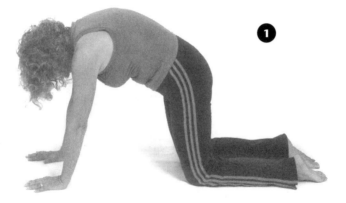

1

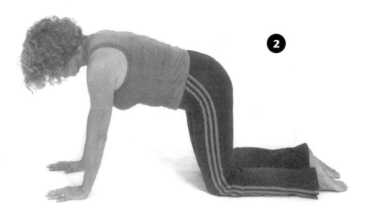

2

For this stretch, try listening to some relaxing music.

STARTING POSITION: Lie on a mat, with your head on a pillow if needed. Focus on breathing slowly in and out through your nose.

1 Reach your arms as far back as is comfortable. Lengthen your legs as far as is possible. Try to make your body as long as possible while breathing in a comfortable fashion. Remember to focus on your breath.

starting position

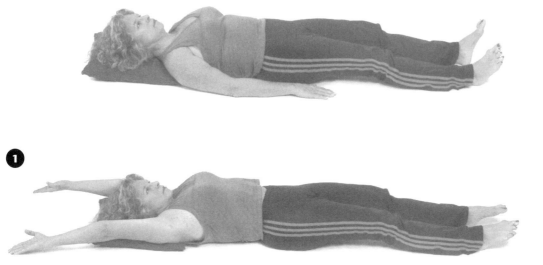

index

other books by ulysses press

WEIGHTS FOR 50+: BUILDING STRENGTH, STAYING HEALTHY AND ENJOYING AN ACTIVE LIFESTYLE

Dr. Karl Knopf, $14.95

Designed to meet the unique needs of the 50+ person, the carefully modified stretches in this book are easy to learn and safe to perform at any age.

YOGA FOR 50+: MODIFIED POSES & TECHNIQUES FOR A SAFE PRACTICE

Richard Rosen, $14.95

As baby boomers pass age 50, problems with knees, ankles and backs are leading them into lower-impact forms of fitness. Tailored specifically for this burgeoning population, *Yoga for 50+* offers a straightforward approach that makes it easy to learn yoga at any age.

PILATES PERSONAL TRAINER BACK STRENGTHENING WORKOUT: ILLUSTRATED STEP-BY-STEP MATWORK ROUTINE

Michael King and Yolande Green, $9.95

The easy starter program in this workbook teaches Pilates exercises that are appropriate for strengthening the back in a safe and healthy manner.

PILATES PERSONAL TRAINER GETTING STARTED WITH STRETCHING: ILLUSTRATED STEP-BY-STEP MATWORK ROUTINE

Michael King and Yolande Green, $9.95

Ideal for beginners or older people, the specially designed Pilates exercises in this book offer a gentle workout of light strength movements and key stretches.

THE PILATES PRESCRIPTION FOR BACK PAIN: A COMPREHENSIVE PROGRAM FOR DEVELOPING AND MAINTAINING A HEALTHY BACK

Lynne Robinson, Helge Fisher and Paul Massey, $14.95

While Pilates has recently become popular as a fitness trend, this book details the self-care program that applies the Pilates principles physical therapists have been using for decades to end back pain.

WEIGHT-BEARING WORKOUTS FOR WOMEN: EXERCISES FOR SCULPTING, STRENGTHENING & TONING

Yolande Green, $12.95

Weight training is the fastest, most effective way to lose fat, improve muscle tone and strengthen bones. This workbook shows just how easy it is for women at any age to get started with weights.

To order these books call 800-377-2542 or 510-601-8301, fax 510-601-8307, e-mail ulysses@ulyssespress.com, or write to Ulysses Press, P.O. Box 3440, Berkeley, CA 94703. All retail orders are shipped free of charge. California residents must include sales tax. Allow two to three weeks for delivery.

about the author

KARL KNOPF has been involved with the health and fitness of the disabled and older adults for almost 30 years. A consultant on numerous National Institutes of Health grants, Knopf has served as advisor to the PBS exercise series "Sit and Be Fit," and to the State of California on disabilities issues. He is a frequent speaker at conferences and has written several textbooks and articles. Knopf is president of the Fitness Educators of Older Adults Association. He also coordinates the Fitness Therapist Program at Foothill College in Los Altos Hills, California.

acknowlegdments

A special thanks goes to Ashley Chase for her vision and for making this book happen. Sincere appreciation goes to Lily Chou and Claire Chun for their attention to detail. Another thought of appreciation goes to our models Phyllis Ritchie, Mike O'Meara and Vivian Gunderson for their patience and efforts. Lastly, my appreciation goes to Robert Holmes for capturing the essence of the stretch.